THE

NEW SYSTEM

OF

EDUCATING HORSES

INCLUDING

INSTRUCTIONS ON FEEDING, WATERING, ETC.

ALSO

HOW SHOEING SHOULD BE DONE;

WITH

SIMPLE PRACTICAL TREATMENT FOR DISEASES.

ILLUSTRATED.

INCLUDING A

LARGE NUMBER OF VALUABLE RECIPES

NOT BEFORE PUBLISHED.

BY D. MAGNER.

☞ This work is written by the Author for the use of his Subscribers.

Ninth Edition, Revised and Enlarged.

BUFFALO:
WARREN, JOHNSON & CO., PRINTERS.

1870.

TO PURCHASERS.

PREFACE.

THE present (ninth) edition of my book will be found by far the most practical and valuable of any I have yet published on the education, *reformation*, care, breeding and diseases of the Horse. Since my former edition was issued, I have had a large experience in the treatment of diseases—have spent considerable time and money in studying with the best veterinary practitioners in this country to obtain the latest and best methods of treating all the common forms of diseases of horses which are here given. The Medical Department of this work will be found particularly valuable, as in it are given remedies and simple treatment for diseases, many of which have never been given to the public, and will be found invaluable. The success and satisfaction with which my previous editions have been received by my former patrons and pupils, gives me assurance that the many new and valuable features contained in this work will be duly appreciated.

D. MAGNER.

☞ Inquiries for this book, or concerning other business, should be addressed to D. Magner, Jamestown, Chautauqua County, N. Y. Price of book, $5.00.

EDUCATION OF HORSES.

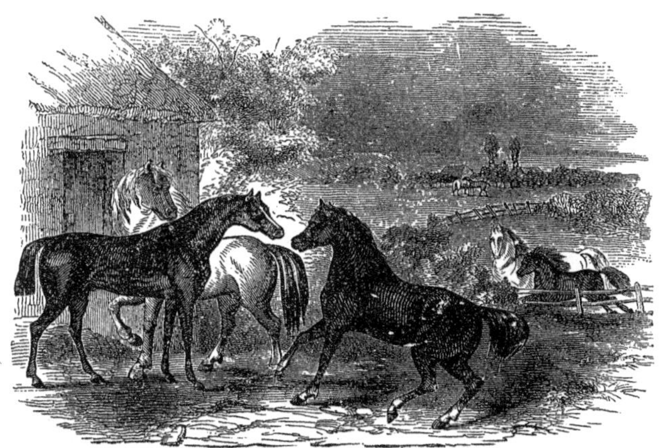

The Horse, by nature, is averse to the control of man, and, of course, knows nothing of the various ways by which he is made to serve the wants of man, except as he is taught.

The Theory *of subjection and management* which has been explained and illustrated to you in my class, however valuable and effective it may seem, can prove so to you only to the degree that you are patient, careful and prudent in its application, and with the hope of being able to aid you still further in correcting some of the grave faults in common practice, I wish to call your attention to a few of the common causes of trouble and failure arising from ignorance of the peculiarities of disposition in horses, as well as imprudence in their management, which should be very carefully guarded against. It must be admitted that our present THEORY, both for general and special resistance, is by far the most scientific and practical that has yet been discovered or brought to notice, and that we can now produce results in the subjection of horses, which were regarded as impossible a few years ago. We have shown how easy it is to control the most powerful horse, and how readily the most vicious animal will yield perfect obedience to every command when properly treated.

But these and all other *principles* are only *rules*, by the use of which certain results are to be secured, and their chief value in practice must depend upon the judgment used in applying them.

The horse has an intellectual, as well as a physical nature, and both are governed by fixed laws. He is an animal of great strength and acute sensibilities, and since it is through the *sensibilities* that the mind is excited to action in calling the strength into play, it is highly important that the nervous system should not be exposed to influences which would excite its undue action, and tend to increase resistance when once aroused.

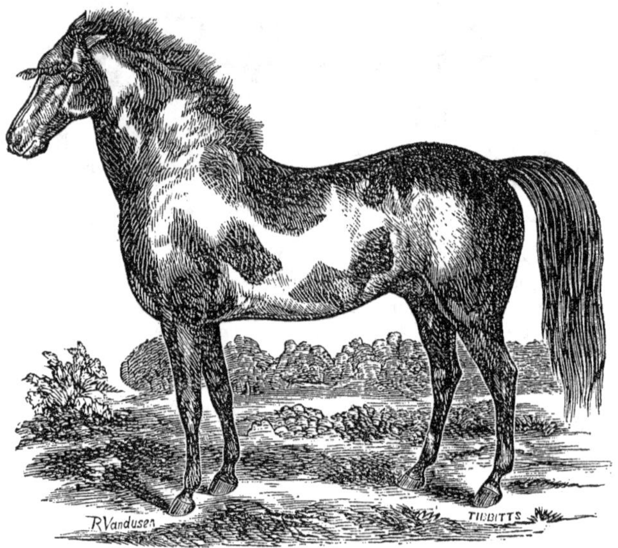

TOMMY—one of Prof. Magner's noted trained horses—the best trick pony in the world.

The mind, or BRAIN, controls the actions of the animal, and it is to this that our efforts must be directed, as the key through which success is to be achieved in training and educating the horse. It is through the brain that the horse understands and obeys, and it is by subjecting the brain, or nervous system to bad impressions that resistance or fear is excited. If fear is excited and the will aroused in securing obedience, the resistance of the animal is stimulated, the legitimate authority and control of the driver weakened or neutralized, and the necessity for force greatly increased. If, however, physical resistance is overcome without arousing the passions or creating fear, no resistance being excited, obedience is easily secured. It should therefore be the first and constant care with every one, as it is one of the great conditions of success, to guard against causes of excitement, which always increase the difficulties, not only by so confusing the mind that it cannot act clearly, but by increasing the amount of resistance which it is so important to prevent.

The physical powers of man are so inferior to those of the horse that controlling him by mere force is out of the question, nor is it necessary. The superiority of mind over matter has been fully demonstrated. We find, by studying the horse's weak points, and taking him at a disadvantage, the impression can be made upon his mind that man's strength is superior to his, and when once he is thoroughly convinced that resistance on his part is entirely useless, this impression answers the same end for all practical purposes, as if man were really the stronger party. We have already shown you how this impression may easily be made, and in the reformation of horses with confirmed bad habits, this is the first point to be gained; but great care and good judgment is necessary, or there is danger of exciting renewed and desperate resistance, sometimes producing a reckless disregard of all restraint, bordering on insanity, or a stupid indifference, which is quite as difficult to overcome.

As soon as the horse yields to the treatment and submits quietly to what is required, we must hasten to secure the coöperation of his affections by kindness, and by giving him something which he likes. This course must be continued, rewarding for obedience and punishing in the way which you have been shown, for disobedience, until the character becomes fixed. This is important, and must never be forgotten.

Many of the characteristics of man have their counterpart in the horse, and we also find a similar diversity of organization. As in man, so also in the horse. The more the lower, coarser, or animal characteristics predominate, or the more the bad nature is excited, the more unreliable and obstinate the character, and the more difficulty will be had in securing obedience.

Thê grand point to be attained is to overcome the animal's natural opposition to restraint, and render his *will* entirely subservient to that of his master, and the great lesson which must be thoroughly impressed upon the mind of the horse is that "disobedience will be punished with pain, but obedience will be rewarded with kindness. The *general theory* and principles by which this is to be done have been sufficiently illustrated to you, and it is my purpose to give in this book only such suggestions and instructions as will enable you to apply my system successfully to the various cases and different subjects necessary in the training and subjection of horses.

From the very commencement, I would caution you against pounding, kicking, yelling and jerking your horse under any circumstances, as such treatment can only irritate and confuse the animal. You must be very patient and thorough in first getting the horse to understand what you wish him to do, taking great care not to excite his fear or resistance, as that will surely involve you in a contest for the mastery, which should be avoided if possible; for, though you may gain the victory, saying nothing of other dangers, the probabilities are ten to one that the *disposition* of your horse will suffer in the struggle. Remember, if you would have kind and reliable horses you must cultivate the better part of their natures, inducing obedience by kindness, without arousing the bad nature, and continue this treatment carefully and patiently, until prompt obedience to your every command becomes a *habit* firmly fixed.

Importance of Uniformity in Language.

Horses cannot understand the meaning of language except so far as associated with actions. To teach a colt to stop at the word "*whoa*," we must first pull upon the halter or bridle at the same time that we give the command, and continue to associate this action with the word until he will obey the word without the action. In the same manner we must teach the meaning of "*go on*," or any other signal to advance, by first using a motion of the hand or a touch of the whip in connection with the command. So the meaning of the word "*back*," and all other words used to express commands, must be carefully and thoroughly taught, *one thing at a time*, until clearly understood. Since the horse cannot obey two commands at once, and has not the power of reason, it seems as if the necessity of being *uniform in language* when addressing the horse, would be felt and appreciated by every one. That is, always use the *same words* in giving the *same command.* Do not say *whoa*, when you wish your horse to *go on;* or *go on*, or *get up*, when you mean *stop;* but always say just what you mean, and then require your horse to do it promptly. Have a certain word or signal for every different command, and always use that and no other. Carelessness or irregularity in giving your commands will make your horse careless in obeying you. Now it is a common fault with most men, in training and using their horses, to talk and act so carelessly in managing them, that it is absolutely impossible for the best trained horses to understand or obey their commands. Of course it is not intentional, and is the result of thoughtlessness rather than lack of judgment. To illustrate, the word "*whoa*" is the generally accepted signal for a horse to *stop* when he is going ahead, and it is evident that if used when the horse is not moving, or for a different purpose, the word loses the force of its meaning, or has no significance whatever. But how many men cry *whoa, whoa*, when they merely wish their horse to go slower, stop shying, change from a trot to a walk, stop pulling at the halter, hold up the head, cease gnawing a post or the fence, stop shaking the head or switching the tail to relieve himself from the annoyance of troublesome flies, and a dozen other things which a horse does so frequently. The same word, more or less sharply uttered, greets the horse on nearly all occasions.

No wonder that the best disposed horse should fail to obey a command which is used for so many different purposes, and should finally become regardless of words which thus become as meaningless to him as Chinese or Choctaw.

Another foolish habit of many drivers which should be avoided, is that of commonly speaking to their horses in a loud or harsh tone of voice. For all ordinary purposes the voice should be rather low and mild, but clear and distinct, and the horse should be taught that when a command is given more sharply and with greater force, he is to obey with so much the more energy and promptness, and unless every word and action used in giving commands, and the degree of force with which they are given, all have a definite and fixed meaning, the horse cannot understand and obey with certainty and readiness.

In training horses, too much must not be attempted at a time. The lessons should be short but *thorough*, always encouraging obedience by kindness and little presents of apples, or something that the animal likes. Special care must be taken to thus caress and reward a sensitive, high spirited and courageous horse, particularly after he has resisted control, and been *forced* to yield.

Extremes of Intelligence and Disposition.

In studying animal nature, we find a general law that the larger and more active the brain, the more intelligence and docility is exhibited; and the smaller and more sluggish the brain, the less intelligence is possessed, and the more determined and active the resistance to control. Consequently we have great extremes and all intermediate modifications of disposition and character, according to the quality and amount of brain and the different predominating faculties. Each type of character is in harmony with this law, in the wild and more savage of the lower animals, as well as those of the domestic classes. We not unfrequently find marked extremes of disposition, even in the same family. For instance, one dog is a model of docility and obedience, while another is surly, cross and savage. In almost every herd of farm animals will be found one more wild or vicious than the others. One cow, one ox or mule is more timid, or ugly, or difficult and dangerous to manage than the rest; and by a similar law we find these various dispositions accompanied by greater or less degrees of vitality,—it being usually the case that those naturally wild and vicious animals are much more hardy and enduring than others.

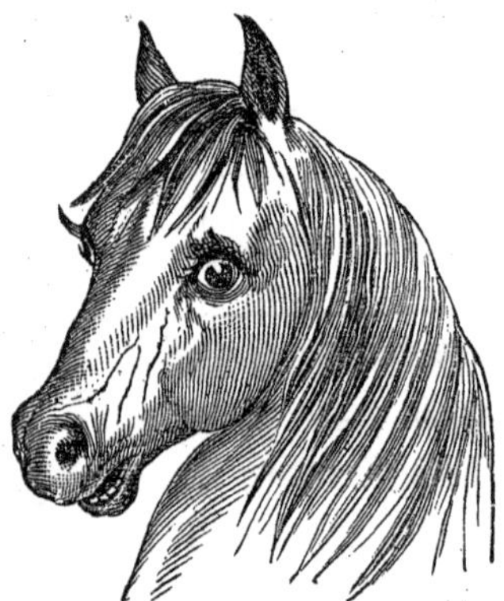
Intelligent and Gentle.

The Horse affords perhaps the best illustration of the diversity of these characteristics. We find that in proportion as there is predominance of the lower and more savage characteristics of animal nature, there is stubbornness of character and power of endurance; and to the degree that animal intelligence and fine sensibility are in excess of the coarse and stubborn traits, there will be tractableness and docility—though perhaps the hardiness and vitality may be somewhat less, yet this is not necessarily the case.

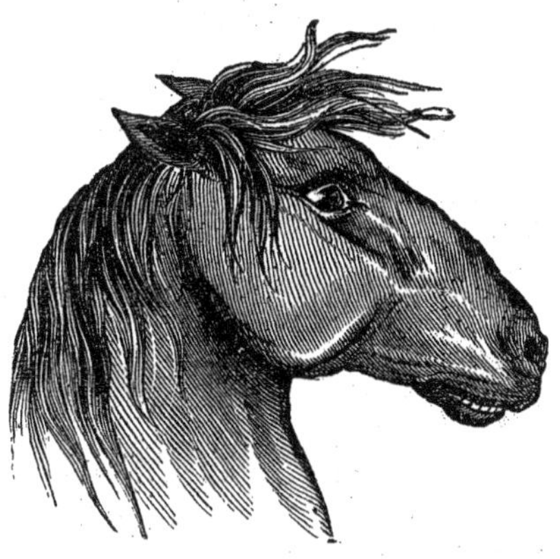
Dull and Treacherous.

The lama, having but little of this coarse nature, will not bear abuse, but will lie down discouraged and die, if overloaded and not relieved. The camel, of a less sensitive type, will toil patiently and nobly under the heaviest burdens, meekly submitting to almost any extreme of abuse. The ass, mule and mustang, having a larger share of the combative disposition, are more obstinate and willful, and are usually more difficult to manage.

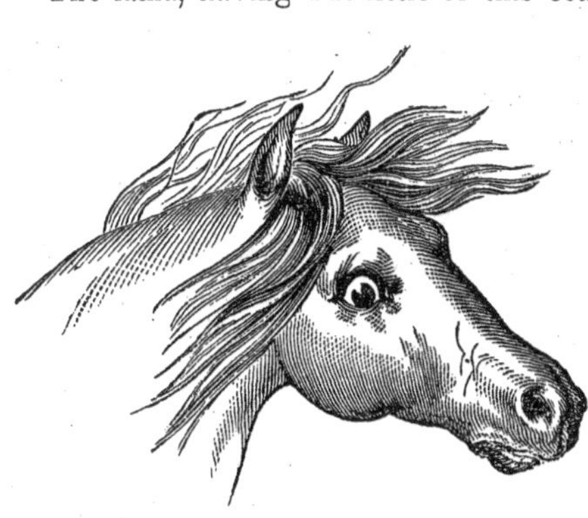
Sensitive and Flighty.

Where there is great predisposition to resistance, more vitality and endurance may be anticipated, but proportionably more skill and judgment will be necessary to secure obedience and docility. This is also true with regard to other animals. Those of a nervous temperament, with but little of the coarse nature, do not need the whip, and will most readily yield obedience to kind and gentle treatment, while those of high courage and strong will, resist control with greater violence and more obstinate energy. The slow, cold-blooded, dull horse, may work kind and gentle from the first time he is harnessed, while the quick, warm-blooded, sensitive horse, is usually nervous and excitable, and must be "worked in" gradually, and managed with more skill and patience to insure perfect submission to the restraint of harness and wagon. This class of horses, more frequently found among thoroughbreds, when fully aroused or greatly excited by fear, are terribly reckless and desperate in their resistance, and require not only very careful, but *very thorough* treatment, and must be made to yield *prompt obedience* to the control of the bit and every word of command.

Indications of Character.

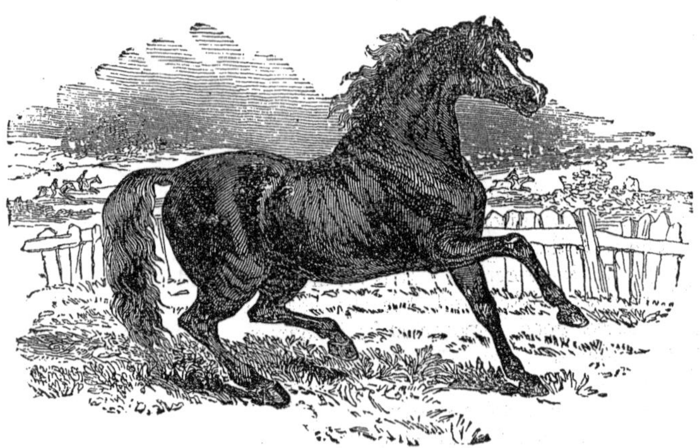

Fiery—Needs watching.

Character, in its general features, is indicated by certain peculiarities. The size, color, coat, shape and size of head, eye and ear, expression of countenance and density of texture, are each an *index* of greater or less significance. Size alone is not a certain indication of strength, but must be taken in connection with quality of limb, form of build, and texture of muscle.

Compact form, strong limb and heavy muscle indicate great strength, and combined with a fine dense texture, denotes activity and great endurance. A large, prominent, bold, eager, but mild and pleasant eye, full, broad forehead, distance short from eye to ear, ears short, tapering and active, indicate great docility and intelligence, while small, round eyes, set well into the head, or eyelids heavy, forehead narrow, long from eye to ear, ears long and flabby, or drooping, indicate a mean, treacherous disposition. Between these extremes there are almost unlimited modifications, developing new phases of character, which call for more or less different treatment in the efforts at training or subjection. To the practiced eye, the exact type of temperament or disposition becomes at once perceptible from these and other peculiarities in the expression of countenance, density of texture, shape of head, size, color and expression of eye, and general appearance.

Rules and Care in Breeding.

There are many remote causes which greatly affect the character of the horse that deserve the serious consideration of the intelligent horseman, and without a knowledge of which there cannot be a correct understanding of the subject, and every effort at breeding must be more or less uncertain, and perhaps unsatisfactory in its results. However apparently trifling first causes may appear in themselves, it is certain that they often lead to consequences which the most careful and thorough subsequent treatment will partially or wholly fail to overcome. It is an inviolate law of nature that "*like produces like*," and it is therefore evident that to raise good horses good horses must be bred from. This is not only true in regard to size, form, soundness and quality of texture, but in disposition. As much care should be taken in selecting horses for *good disposition* as for size, speed, form and strong constitution. In studying causes which positively affect the character and disposition, if we would get at the source we must go back to the time the parents were brought together, and ascertain the condition of their nervous systems, for it is undoubtedly true that the condition of the *sire* or *dam* at the time of connection, and the condition in which the mare is kept, and her treatment during gestation, have a powerful influence upon the character of the colt. If a stallion of the most gentle character is greatly irritated and angry when used to the mare, so marked is the effect of the excitement, that the colt is almost sure to prove of a bad, irritable, temper. If the mare is subjected to a sudden and extreme shock of fear while in foal, the colt is very liable to prove nervous, irritable and unreliable in character.

Bad Effects of Fright.

In other ways, marked extremes of viciousness, approaching sometimes almost to insanity, may be produced by more direct and perceptible causes. To illustrate this, I will refer to one out of many instances which have come under my own observation. A three years old colt, which was noted for gentleness, it having been raised a pet, was allowed to run at large and trespassed upon a neighbor's premises. Dogs, chasing and shouting, had lost all influence in keeping the colt away, so, in a spirit of vexation, the boys tied a tin pan to the colt's tail and then set the dogs after it. At first the colt did not seem to notice the pan, but when pressed by the dogs, and the pan began to rattle and pound against his heels, alarm was excited. The most frantic efforts to get away from the terrible object were resorted to, by kicking and running, until the colt was exhausted, and so powerful was the effect upon the nervous system, that ever after the stirring of anything near or touching the hind parts, would excite the greatest fear and most reckless kicking. The fear thus produced became involuntary; the nervous system was deranged, and the colt spoiled. No matter what may be the cause of the excitement, if greatly frightened, the effect upon the nervous system is always the same, and the greatest care should be taken to guard against causes of fright or unusual excitement, especially in colts. The most careless observer cannot fail to have noticed that when horses which are afraid of a robe, an umbrella, a top wagon, the cars, or anything else, are at some time suddenly frightened by the object, break loose and get away, the impression of fear becomes so strong, that that object is ever after a source of the greatest terror to them. Once breaking loose, running away and kicking, or in any way successfully resisting control, under such circumstances, leads to the habit becoming fixed. It is the brain by which the animal understands and is influenced, and it is the *effect* produced directly or indirectly upon the brain, by rousing the fears and passions, which excites resistance. The efforts should therefore be so applied as to weaken or neutralize that effect by diverting the attention and winning the action of the mind in an opposite direction. This end you have seen, can most easily be attained by my treatment, and with prudence and careful management the worst horses can usually be reformed by my system in a short time.

Whipping Dangerous.

I would caution those who train or use horses upon another point, viz.: that of exciting the ill will of the animal. Many think they are doing finely, and are proud of their success in horse training by means of severe whipping, or otherwise rousing and stimulating the passions, and then, from necessity, *crushing* the will, through which the resistance is prompted. No mistake can be greater than this, and there is nothing that so fully exhibits the ability, judgment and skill of the real horseman, as the care and tact displayed in winning, instead of repelling the action of the mind. Although it may be necessary to use the whip sometimes, it should always be applied judiciously, and great care should be taken not to rouse the passions, or excite the *will* to obstinacy. The legitimate and proper use of the whip is calculated to operate upon the sense of *fear* almost entirely. The affections and better nature must be appealed to in training a horse, as well as in training a child. A reproof given may be intended for the good of the child, but, if only the *passions* are excited, the effect is depraving and injurious. This is a vital principle, and can be disregarded in the management of sensitive, courageous horses, only at the imminent risk of spoiling them. I have known many horses of a naturally gentle character, to be spoiled by being whipped once; and one horse that was made *vicious* by being struck with a whip *once*, while standing in his stall.

I have referred to these instances to show the *danger* of rough treatment, and the effects which may be easily produced by ill usage, especially with fine blooded horses and those of a highly nervous temperament. Many other cases might be cited, as such are by no means uncommon. Sensitive horses should never be left after they have been excited by the whip or other means, until calmed down by rubbing or patting the head and neck, and giving apples, sugar, or something of which the animal is fond. Remember the whip must be used with great care, or it is liable to do mischief, and may cause irreparable injury.

Courage in Handling Horses.

Many men boast that they "are not afraid of any living horse," &c. To a really experienced horseman such assertions betray ignorance and inexperience. Very many of the most lamentable accidents that occur with horses are the result of this foolhardy imprudence. It is almost impossible to convince a man who has never been run away with, that a horse *could* run away while *he* held the reins, or that he *cannot* drive a kicker safely by any care that can be used; and when such men are run away with, or have a horse kick the wagon to pieces and get away, they will declare that they can drive and manage any horse but *that one.*

Any horse that has learned to resist the bit successfully, *cannot* be held or safely controlled by the reins when under great excitement, and it is idle for *any* man to pretend that it can be done. I have found hundreds of horses which would run away every time they were driven, regardless of the most severe bits, though pulled upon by several men. I have seen horses that, on a walk, would pull two and even four men, by the reins, though tugging and pulling as they pleased. Of course it is the most senseless imprudence to talk of driving and holding such horses, when there is almost *certainty* of being unable to retain control should the animal become excited.

While it is highly important to appear fearless and confident when approaching and handling horses, it is not to be assumed that a horse will not bite, strike or kick, because courage is shown. An Irishman, who supposed a horse would not attack or injure him if he would stand still and show no fear, walked into the enclosure of a vicious stallion. The horse rushed upon him, bit and struck him down, and it was with the greatest difficulty that he was rescued, even at the cost of a broken arm, three ribs and a leg, with serious internal injuries.

I once encountered a terribly vicious mare, and having purposely been kept in ignorance of her bad character, I went into the yard without sufficient precaution, and had to jump for my life to get away from her. When she rushed for me

I instantly saw that escape was my only alternative, and sprang head foremost over the high enclosure. It was a trick to defeat me, as all my *would be* pupils laughed, and for the first time I discovered that they were all over head and out of all possible danger. This was one of the most desperate and dangerous specimens of the horse that I ever saw. She would run at a man with all the ferocity of a mad dog, and would no doubt have bit and trampled me under foot in a moment, could she have got hold of me. But in thirty minutes I made her perfectly gentle, and safe for any one to approach and handle.

The horse always reveals his intentions by the action of his ears and expression of his eye, as plainly as could be done in words. In approaching a horse, the notice should be carefully directed to the head for an understanding of the intentions. If danger is discernible, and is not too imminent, stand still. It will not do to show, by the expression of the features or faltering of the voice, that fear is felt. When a bad horse *must* be encountered, especially if a stallion, the eye must be kept steadily on that of the horse, and the *will* must be inflexible. Adroitness and firmness in diverting the attention, will hold some horses of a dangerous character in check, when the least exhibition of weakness or fear would precipitate a calamity. Some horses, stallions in particular, seem to read the feelings of a groom, or any one handling them, as plainly as could a man, and any indication of timidity will encourage them to resistance. Whatever the feelings or apprehension of danger, there must be no evidence of fear exposed in the language or actions. There is a peculiar acuteness of perception acquired by long experience and observation, that cannot be explained, but which enables one at a glance to see how far it is safe to approach and handle a horse of a dangerous character. Indeed, I do not know of any profession or calling which requires more acuteness of perception, or firmness and judgment, in directing and controlling the efforts, than that of the professional horseman. Discretion is sometimes the better part of valor, and the courage shown should always be according to circumstances. No one should recklessly expose himself to the fury of a vicious horse, and when necessary to handle such, it should be done with the greatest caution and judgment, always taking care to first confine the horse in some way, until the bridle or other means of control can be securely attached. It is well, perhaps, to remind in this connection, that the subjection and successful reformation of some horses will often call for much resource of prudence and skill. Horses having small, round eyes, set well into the head, or heavy eyelids, gray or sorrel color, denote the hardest cases. They will sometimes show the obstinate recklessness of a bull dog. Young horses, too, are often the most trying. Do not be discouraged because such are obstinately persistent. My principles of subjection will enable, with anything like ordinary effort, *absolute control* of any horses. First, if you anticipate the animal to be plucky and determined, work quick, until there is submission, putting through the regular routine of *subjection.* When you have cases of this kind, if possible make your point before the horse can become warmed up to any considerable degree, as greatly heating the blood blunts the sensibilities and stimulates resistance to an extraordinary degree, and instead of the subject working in easily and gently when attempted to be driven in harness, he will be more likely to resist restraint. Skill and tact in this will add very much to your success in working the horse into good character. The *second method* of subjection is your principal reliance, in extreme cases. If necessary, disabling in driving, by the foot trap, is often useful. After making your point, hold it by driving and handling until the animal is entirely cool and gentle. The impression should be fixed by rewarding liberally with sugar and salt, &c., when there is submission. Remember the character is not always set and made reliable by the animal being made to yield, and drive gently once or twice. Handle cautiously for a few times, expecting resistance, and ready to combat it until the character is made reliable. This prudence is the more necessary if the animal is valuable.

Reference to the different heads in another part of this book will give details for the proper management of different peculiarities of disposition and habit. In studying the laws of equine subjection and education, many striking truths are forced upon the mind. The wisdom displayed by the Creator in adapting the different domestic animals to the wants of man, the ease with which they can be subdued and controlled, when subjected to proper and reasonable treatment, is truly wonderful, and the inevitable consequences of every act of imprudence committed in their management is strikingly clear and positive, reminding us that it is not only our duty, but economy and wisdom in us to *correct* the errors of imprudence and ignorance which have been so long and so extensively practiced by the masses. This duty addresses itself at once to the reason and all the higher faculties of the mind, and, in its true sense, is in every way inspiring to a higher feeling of responsibility and elevation of character.

☞ If the owner wishes, he is at liberty to read the foregoing part of this work to others, it not being in any way an infringement upon the secrecy imposed.

TRAINING THE WILD COLT.

The opposition and resistance of a colt is *natural*, and is induced by fear and ignorance of what is required of him. Colts of a highly sensitive or positive nature will often resist being handled or controlled, with the most reckless perversity. When much obstinacy is anticipated or shown, the first thing to be accomplished is to overcome such sensibility and resistance as will ensure safety to the operator in handling the animal as he desires. If this point be thoroughly made, the colt will be sufficiently plastic and submissive to ensure safety in his management and certainty of control. To produce such results, much prudence and skill is often necessary, and the reader must bear in mind that his success in training and educating horses will depend upon the discrimination and judgment with which his efforts are adapted in applying my *Theory of Management.*

If possible, the operator should have a good room or training yard, about twenty-five or thirty feet square, or even larger. See that all causes of injury are removed, and get the colt into this enclosure very quietly; if he is wild and nervous, see that no hens, dogs, etc., are in the room. Say to your friends, it is necessary to your success, and is a condition of your instruction, that you must be *alone.*

Of course the colt must first be haltered. If not very wild, this will not be difficult to do. But if very wild or vicious, this may be difficult and perhaps dangerous, and you should always carefully guard against injury to yourself as well as your horse, and at the same time you may accomplish your object just as surely, if not as easily. Take a light pole ten or twelve feet in length, or as much longer as you can use to advantage, if the colt is very wild or dangerous, and drive two nails into it, about eight inches apart, the first about an inch from the end, with the heads bent a little outward from each other. Take a common rope halter with a running noose, pull the part which slips through the noose back about two feet, and hang the part that goes over the head upon the nails on the end of your pole nicely, keeping hold of the hitching part, which must be as long as your pole. Your halter is now so spread and hung upon the stick as to be easily put on to the head. If the colt is not excited or frightened, as you extend the halter towards him he will reach out his nose to smell and examine it, and while he is gratifying his curiosity in this way, you can bring the slack part under his jaw and raise the pole high enough to bring the halter over and back of the ears, when, by turning the stick half way round, the halter will drop from it upon the head. This will frighten the colt a little and cause him to run from you, but this will only cause the slack part passing back of the jaw to be pulled up, and the halter will be securely adjusted.

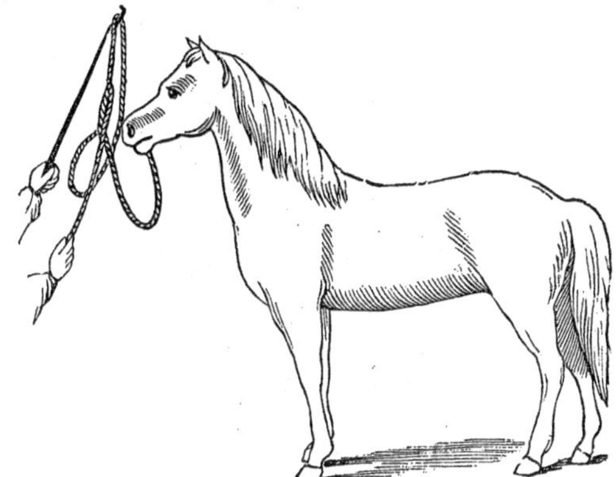

Haltering the Colt.

Being haltered, the colt must now be taught to submit to its restraints and yield to control. Take a position at the side of the colt, on a line with his shoulder, but at some distance, and give a quick, strong pull towards you, instantly letting loose on the halter until you get the same position again. You have the greatest advantage from this position, and by adroitly following it, never attempting to pull when he runs back or from you, the colt will soon learn to yield to the slightest pull in that direction, and will follow your every movement *on that side* without pulling scarcely at all. Should you pull slow and steady, he will learn to resist and pull against you, and might throw himself down; but this you will avoid by giving a quick pull, bringing him towards you, and letting loose instantly. As soon as he will yield and come to you promptly on one side, get on the other side and repeat the lesson in the same manner, until the colt will follow you readily and quickly on either side without pulling. Be careful not to pull ahead until there is prompt submission sidewise. You can then gradually pull a little more on a line with the body until the colt will come to you promptly in any direction, and yield readily to the slightest pull upon the halter. If the colt is intelligent, and of a quick, tractable disposition, he will soon learn this lesson thoroughly; but if very young, or of a slow, sulky disposition, great resistance is likely to be shown. If the resistance is very obstinate or reckless in character, you must resort at once to a *thorough course of subjection*, which will soon compel obedience. This you have been taught how to do; and here I will only say that in most cases with colts, a short course by the *second method* is sufficient, always being careful not to tie too short. With older horses, and with colts of certain dispositions, the *first method* is usually very effective.

Whenever there is submission you should encourage and fix it by appealing at once to the affections. Rub the head, pat the neck and scratch the mane and tail until all excitement and irritation subside. The eye will now be mild in expression, and there is an apparent indifference to being handled. A coarse, harsh or loud voice is terribly irritating to a sensitive or spirited horse or colt, and must by all means be held in check. Speak in a gentle and natural tone, and let your voice be softened by kind expression, for it will do much toward securing the confidence of the animal and repressing his fear. With some colts it will be necessary to repeat the lesson in leading two or three times, to fix the point of prompt obedience. In every case the lesson should be made very thorough.

Hitching.

When the colt will lead kindly and promptly, he may next be taught to stand hitched. To prevent the possibility of his learning to pull at the halter, take a piece of strong cord, about a third of an inch in diameter, sufficiently long when doubled to be a little shorter than the halter when hitched, and tie it in the following manner: Find the middle and put it under the tail; bring both ends forward, cross and twist them three or four times over on the back, do the same in front of the breast, pass them through the ring of the halter

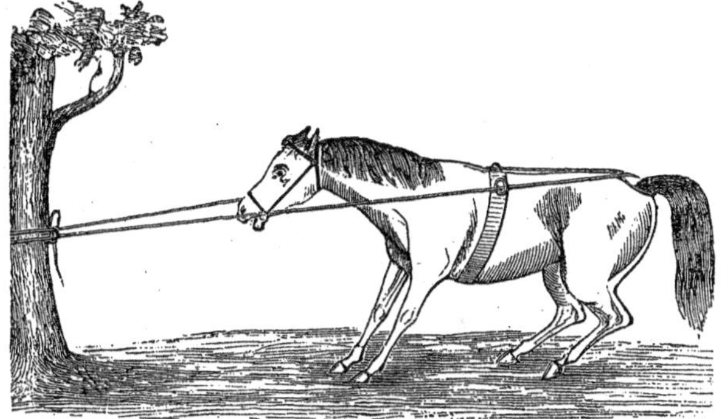

Hitching.

and tie to the manger or post. Hitch in this way until the colt refuses to pull back, even if frightened a little, and after two or three days the halter can be depended upon with safety.

Bitting

Is the next step in educating the colt, and implies not only teaching the colt to submit to the restraint and control of the bit, but giving as much style to the carriage of the head and neck as the form and temper of the animal will bear. If the bitting is imperfectly done, the horse may acquire habits of resisting the bit, such as lugging upon the check, pulling too hard on the bit, pulling on one rein, refusing to back, etc. To do this thoroughly and properly may seem to be a difficult task, but it is a simple matter and very easily accomplished. The colt's mouth should first become accustomed to the bit. To do this, put on a common bridle with a smooth snaffle bit, without reins, and allow him to go as he pleases, in a yard or field, for half an hour or more, which may be repeated once or twice. Next put on surcingle with check and side reins, buckling the reins at first so long as to bring but little restraint upon the mouth. After being on thirty or forty minutes, remove, and at each repetition buckle the reins a little shorter, until the desired style of carriage is secured. The colt should have at least one lesson each day, but never more than two, as it is better to proceed slowly and thoroughly.

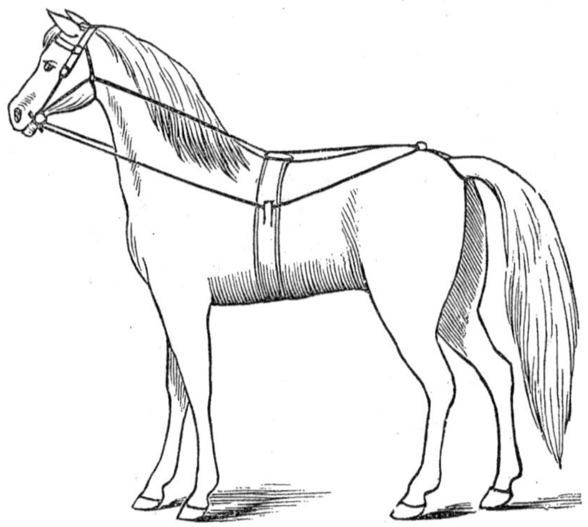

Bitting the Colt.

It seems needless to introduce details of a bitting harness. Any simple construction of the ordinary kind will answer very well, and the style is so generally understood that a description here is unnecessary. The object being to bring such restraint upon the bit that the head will be held up and back most naturally and easily, without giving freedom to the head except in the direction of the reins. Care should be taken to have the throat latch loose enough to not press upon the throat when the colt is checked up, and the gag-runners should be well up near the ears. Care must be taken not to bring too much restraint upon the bit by buckling the reins too short at first, as it is liable to excite such resistance that the colt will rear up and fall over backwards, which would be almost certain to result in death. Colts should not be checked up too long at a time, as it becomes tiresome, and the colt will learn to rest his head upon the bit and thus form the very disagreeable habit of *lugging*. If, however, the colt should fight the restraint of the bit or check, it should be left on till the fit exhausts itself and he shows a disposition to submit to its restraint.

The bitting bridle should not be kept on very long at a time. Short lessons at first, and gradually longer as the mouth becomes hardened by the bit and the colt will bear it without fatigue, is the proper course for bitting in this manner. But simply subjecting the mouth to *this* course of discipline does not teach submission to the restraint of the bit, nor does it cause the horse to throw his head up and back when the reins are pulled upon, as he should; or at least to only a limited extent. Hence it is that many horses acquire a disposition to lug against the bit, throw the head down on the breast, pull sidewise, throw the head forward, or some other peculiar form of resistance in consequence of this imperfect mode of bitting. All these tendencies I easily overcome by the following simple treatment:

After the usual course of bitting is completed, or has been in progress several days or a week, take a piece of cord about eight or ten feet in length, of the common sash or clothes line size, as strong and pliable as you can find. Tie a large hard knot in one end, and about twenty inches from this knot make another tie, passing the knot end around the neck so it will just fit the neck forward of the shoulder. Pass the other end of the cord through both rings of the bit, back of the jaw and back through the loop around the neck, and draw up the slack. Now stand in front of the head, holding the cord tightly with both hands; give a quick, short pull downwards, which will cause the head to be thrown up and back. Repeat this little jerking, downward pull, until the head is given up and back freely at the slightest pull. Now, when the reins are attached to the bit and pulled upon, the restraint is precisely the same as before; and after repeating this lesson a few times, the head will be freely submitted to the control of the bit, and a beautiful carriage of the head secured, even without a check.

Harnessing.

The harness may now be put on, and the next step will be to teach the colt to be guided, right or left, and stopped at pleasure. No attempt should be made to teach the colt to *back*, until he has learned to drive well to wagon; for if first taught to back, there is danger that he will acquire the habit of running back when confused or frightened.

If the colt is sensitive, and you wish to be very thorough, after putting on the harness carefully, you may tie up the tugs and let him run about the yard for half an hour. Now put on the reins and gradually teach him to go ahead, turn right or left, or stop, as you please, by the restraint of the bit. Too much must not be expected of a colt at once, and the trainer should always be careful not to excite the animal, or to get excited himself.

Hitching to Wagon Poles.

If the colt is at all uncertain, it will be policy to work slowly and carefully, as one mismove now may cause serious mischief, by the colt becoming nervous and unmanageable, and, should he be able to resist restraint, will easily cause a loss, by damage to wagon, of from five to fifty dollars. To guard against this, get THREE SLENDER POLES, two of them about twelve feet long each, the third about seven feet in length. Lay down the poles in the form of shafts, the front ends about twenty inches apart, the back ends about six feet apart. Lay the short piece across about six feet six inches from the forward ends, and tie on with pieces of cord. Hitch the colt into these poles, attaching the tugs to the cross pieces by tying with small cord, and drive the colt around until there is perfect submission to them. Driving to poles is an advantageous step, for two reasons: they cause less noise and excitement, and consequently are less likely to cause resistance; and should the horse kick, no damage can result—whereas, one kick against a buggy would be likely to cause serious damage and loss.

Before attempting to drive a colt to the wagon or shafts, all danger of resisting anything striking the heels should be thoroughly overcome by the course of subjection. It is always the safest and best method. Anything like a suitable cart or two-wheeled sulky can be obtained by but few, and the cheapness and ease of constructing poles into the form of shafts will enable any one, at a trifling trouble, by this means to easily supply that want.

In driving to poles or shafts, the horse should be made to submit to touching against the hind parts in every manner possible, without offering resistance. When hitched, let the colt move off moderately, at first, gradually requiring him to go right and left, back against the cross piece, etc. But mind, do not commit the error of making young horses, when first trained to harness, go back too freely, as it leads to the habit of running back at the slightest causes of excitement in front of them. Great care should be taken not to drive the colt too much at first, and at no time sufficient to produce exhaustion. Neither should his strength be taxed too much by driving up or down hill, until he has become accustomed to the noise and restraint of the wagon and learned to use his strength as required. Let his drives be moderate at first, both in gait and distance; about a mile or two on a walk first, gradually increasing the distance as he will bear without fatigue. After he will go nicely on a walk, let him trot a little, gradually letting him out faster and a little further, as nice, smooth pieces of road give opportunity; but be very particular to restrict these little outbursts of speed at first to the limits of a few rods, and never allow the colt to become exhausted. Let him dash out a short distance, then gradually slacken to a walk, speaking kindly and encouragingly as you would if talking to a boy. After a while, let him out again, pushing, perhaps, a little faster and further, being careful not to crowd him to breaking. It must not be expected because your colt is perhaps a good mover, that he will be a *fast trotter*. But if he is a really good stepper, it is so much the more necessary for you to use judgment and prudence in his training. There is usually too much anxiety to try a colt's speed and bottom, and he is often pushed, overdone, and spoiled perhaps, before his powers are half developed.

A colt must not be crowded too much in educating to harness. It is evident that he cannot be expected to submit quietly to the irritation and excitement of harness and wagon, or drive quietly like an old horse, without experience. He must grow into familiarity with these things from usage and contact with them. The trainer must be particularly careful in the outset to overcome all fear from things TOUCHING the HIND LEGS and parts of the body. This lesson must be very thorough, and as each progressive step in educating the colt is attempted, this point must not be lost sight of; and if each successive point is clearly and thoroughly accomplished, patient, careful labor will be rewarded in the possession of a kind, gentle, trusty and well-behaved animal, whose services will always afford pleasure to his owner and driver.

Double Driving.

It is generally the custom to drive the colt at first in harness by the side of a gentle horse accustomed to harness. When this is to be done, the colt should be put on the off side, and to guard against danger, a short strap, with a ring on it, should be put around the fore foot, below the fetlock. Fasten the end of a piece of rope or strap about eight or ten feet long to the ring. Pass the other end over the belly-band of the harness and back to the wagon. The strap is to be held with the reins to insure the utmost control, should the colt become frightened and attempt to break away or kick. The whip should be held over the old horse, to keep him up to the movements of the colt in starting, but the gait should be kept moderate.

In breaking the colt to drive double, after driving well on the off side, he should be reversed to the near side, there being less danger of becoming frightened from getting into or out of the wagon, or of seeing things while being passed to or from the wagon, by being more from view on the off side. To lessen the probabilities of fear and resistance, the off side is preferable at first. The limited understanding of the horse seems to require that the same impressions and understanding should be given of the character and appearance of things forced to his attention on both sides. If not, when driven alone, or on the near side, he may become suddenly frightened by the moving of a robe, umbrella, the rustling of a lady's dress, etc., from that side. (See Causes of Fear.)

Let the driving be moderate, and the load light, and, by all means, if the colt is of a sensitive or nervous temperament, the greatest mildness must be observed. Loud "yelling" or cracking of the whip should not be permitted. A little imprudence of this kind is often the cause of very serious mischief with timid, young horses.

Backing.

After learning to drive well, teach the idea of backing by pulling on the reins steadily, and saying "back." If there is resistance give a quick, sharp, raking pull, which will move the colt by the pain and force of the bit backward, repeating until there is prompt obedience. If there is much resistance put on breaking bit, which will soon secure submission.

Riding.

If the colt is not of a very bad character there will be no resistance to being rode after the first lesson of subjection. If there is, attach a short strap or a piece of rope to the off fore foot, throwing the other end over the back. Take a short hold of this strap with the right hand, while the left grasps the near rein of the bridle firmly. As the head is pulled around, the horse is made to step sidewise, and the instant the foot is relaxed it is held up by the restraint of the right hand on the strap, which is instantly drawn upon. The colt is now on three legs, and unable to resist. Jump lightly on the back, press the feet against the belly and flanks. As there is submission release the foot, taking a firm hold of the reins, which should be held short. Move the colt forward, and as there is an indication of resistance pull upon the strap and reins, which will disable and disconcert the horse from further opposition to being rode. If the colt will not move forward, request an assistant to lead him by the head for a short time. So long as there is any indication of resistance, keep on the strap. One thorough lesson is usually sufficient, though some colts may require a repetition of the lesson.

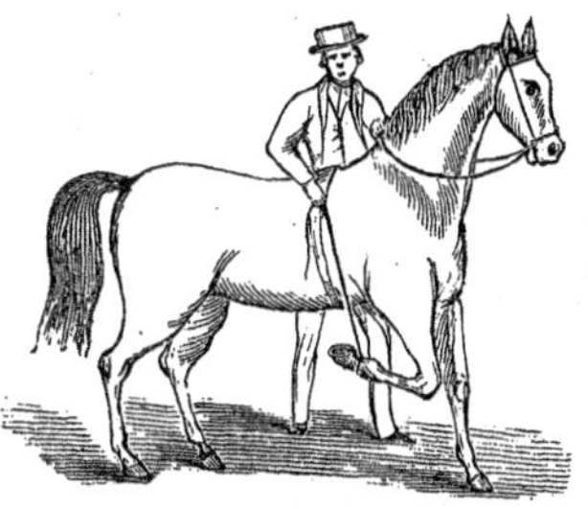
Riding.

When it is desired to mount, let the left hand rest lightly on the mane, a little forward of the withers, holding the reins between the thumb and fingers. Throw the right hand lightly on the back, the body close to the horse. Now spring lightly upward and forward. The instant of doing so, let the right hand glide forward until the elbow strikes the back bone, when the weight of the body is to be instantly balanced upon the right arm, which will enable sufficient strength to make the spring continuous, and the body is easily brought into a sitting posture. This is a slight undertaking, and a little practice will give the ability to mount the highest horses with apparently wonderful ease. To mount on a saddle, stand by the side, a little back of the stirrup, the face exactly towards the horse's head. Take a short hold of the reins between the fingers, grasping into the mane at the same time, put the left foot into the stirrup, throw the right hand over the saddle and press it against the off side, throwing the weight of the body on the left foot, and you can lift yourself into the saddle easily.

Handling the Feet.

If the colt is of an ordinary good disposition this can be done without resorting to special means. Stand well up to the shoulder, put the left hand on the shoulder, pressing forward gently, which will relax the muscles controlling the leg, with the right hand, instantly grasp the foot below the fetlock and lift it up, removing the left hand and bring under the foot to aid the right hand, or wholly liberating the right hand. To handle the hind feet, let the right hand glide gently from the shoulders back to the hip. At the instant it passes the point of the hip, bring the left forward upon the hip. While doing this, the right hand is being glided down the leg gently, until it strikes the fetlock, when the left hand is pressed firmly against the body at the point stated, which will relax the limb, as before, and the foot is easily brought up by the right. At the instant of raising with the right, the left is lowered and passed down the limb on the back part of the fetlock. Or the foot can be raised and lowered a few times with the right hand, while the left balances the body by pressing against the hip until there is perfect submission.

If there is resistance, take up the fore foot, request an assistant to hold it up for you, while he at the same time holds the colt by the halter or bridle. Tie the end of a rope or strap around the hind foot, above the fetlock, at the instant of doing which let the hand glide along to the opposite part, until six or eight feet from the foot. At the same time request the forward foot to be let loose, the assistant holding by the halter. Now pull upon the strap, which will bring the foot forward, and at the instant of attempting to kick, let go, and so repeat until the foot is submitted to the restraint of strap. Then slip behind and pull the foot back, and as before yielding at each effort to kick, let go, until the foot is submitted freely. Now take the foot from the control of the strap to the hand and handle gently.

If there is very determined resistance, tie the end of your long strap around the neck, near the shoulders, pass the other end back between the fore legs, around the hind foot, but under the strap around the neck and draw up on it, at the same time holding him by the bridle or halter. The colt may be frightened and jump to get clear of the restraint. Should he act very much frightened, slack up on the strap until the foot is almost back to its natural position. Then as he will bear, again pull a little shorter, at the same time pulling him round in a circle by the head, until he ceases struggling to get the foot loose. You may now pull the foot farther forward, and hold it as before, until he will stand quietly. Now step back a little and pass the hand down the hind leg. Slap the hand upon the leg a little until there is no resistance, then take it in the hands. If there is no resistance, undo the end of the strap and allow the foot a little more freedom; at the same time while holding the foot by the strap, pass the hand from the hip down the leg quietly, rubbing and caressing until able to take it in the hands.

Handle the opposite legs in the same manner, until there is perfect submission. There is a natural tendency to do nothing more as soon as the feet can be handled, and if there is trouble in shoeing afterwards, it is not assigned to the real cause. It must be borne in mind, that in all cases to insure perfect submission, the feet should be repeatedly handled in the stable or wherever kept, until there is no fear or resistance manifested. This end may not always be accomplished by handling once. The character of the colt is sometimes so sensitive and positive that as much depends upon handling a few times gently after forcing submission, as in the treatment that may be necessary at first.

Fear,

Directly or indirectly, is the principal cause of danger and resistance in horses, and to successfully educate young horses requires that there should be perpetual precaution in preventing such excitement from any cause as would induce fear of any object or sound. The horse's mind, or nervous system is so liable to be thrown out of balance by sudden causes of great fear, that very much of their successful management must depend upon the tact and judgment in preventing such consequences. One of the most remarkable features of this peculiarity, too, is the persistence there is in resisting the object or cause exciting a sense of danger. Thus a robe, umbrella, or other object once exciting an apprehension of danger, is likely to become a source of the greatest terror. When there is the least appearance of an excitable imagination, the most positive sense of control should be fixed upon the understanding, so as to lessen the tendency, and at the same time give power to force obedience to the extreme necessary. The great difficulty in the management of horses predisposed to sensitiveness, or those becoming afraid of some object or causes with which their use requires contact, is want of sufficient power to coerce. I would not imply that gentleness is not an important essential; but it must not be to the mind of the horse the actuating motive, while the fear of disobedience must be so fixed upon the mind, that the disposition to resist control is neutralized. This is the point to make first, if possible. (Which is now seen to be easily done.) Then gently and carefully bring to the understanding a clear conviction of the harmless character of the object or sound, whatever it is. If the colt is wild and sensitive, the first step to be taken is to give him a thorough *course* of *subjection*. If the habit is very bad, it becomes absolutely necessary to do so.

There is in some colts a natural predisposition to extreme sensibility and fear of the most ordinary causes of irritation. A small brain, denoted by a narrow forehead, or a clear, sharp, open, restless eye, indicates this character.

But we see, too, that colts of the very best disposition are easily spoiled by ignorant, imprudent treatment.

It is very remarkable, also, that many colts of the most sensitive and excitable character, by one or two lessons of careful, thorough treatment, become as tractable and obedient as old, gentle horses. I could refer to very many interesting cases in proof of this. One of the most marked in my recent experience, (Oct., 1868,) to which I will refer, was a six year old horse, owned by A. Smawley, of Petroleum Centre, Pa. This horse was of so remarkably wild and desperate a character that he was known by the name of "Wild Pete." He would scringe and jump at the least touch or appearance of anything strange; he would not stand to be cleaned, could not be harnessed, and to attempt putting him in shafts would excite the utmost desperation, jumping and kicking clear of restraint at all hazards. He was one of the most desperate acting horses of the kind I ever saw. Indeed, anything touching him behind, even a touch of a whip, would make him jnmp and kick regardless of consequences. Yet, after subjecting him to two or three energetic lessons of less than an hour each, I could drive him to my buggy with perfect safety, and he could not be made to kick or resist control. So perfectly docile did he become, that he was let for driving in the livery, and has proved a very superior and safe carriage horse. As a rule, however, constitutionally timid horses yield slowly, and require careful as well as thorough treatment.

Colts of the gentlest and apparently most fearless disposition, are often made so nervous and excitable by being once greatly frightened in some way, as to become of the most nervous and dangerous character, or are really *insane* so far as certain particular objects in certain positions are concerned. This is illustrated by the number of otherwise gentle, young horses that are frightened at some particular object, or cannot be driven in harness. When the cause is traced out it will be found in every instance to have been the result of being greatly frightened or excited in some way. Sometimes the most trifling causes will derange the horse in this manner. Even the accidental moving of a piece of white paper will sometimes so excite a previously docile colt, that he will afterwards be a flighty, unreliable animal, always on the alert to jump, and possibly kick at the least appearance of such an object. Incidents of this kind are common to the observation of every one in the least familiar with the peculiarities of equine nature. Now unless the colt is made perfectly obedient and docile, to bear handling and the restraint of harness, and the rattle of the wagon, this being suddenly frightened at some imaginary or trifling cause, is at any moment possible. The first object of the efforts should be to see that every step of progress is made so thoroughly as to preclude such a possibility, which can be easily done by making the colt familiar and submissive to the restraint of the bit, and fearless of the contact and rattle of the wagon, etc., before hitching.

The great difficulty with most people is, they are too harsh and too hasty. They undertake to do, and require more than they have power to enforce, or than the horse is able to understand.

In educating the colt, the rule should be to do and require only so much as he will bear and understand, by commencing slowly and gently repeating, and following up one advantage after another, to the end of inspiring entire disregard of the causes of excitement. The horse's principal mediums of understanding are seeing and feeling with the nose. Through these he examines things new and strange to him. If in approaching the colt you reach out the hand gently, he will smell and feel of it with his nose. Every other means of understanding seems to be subordinate to this, consequently in handling the colt we should always commence at the nose, then gradually work back, as there is submission. The same care should be taken to overcome fear of being handled about the feet, etc. Commence at an insensible part and work to the sensitive. In educating to harness, the same prudence should be exercised by bringing the object to the nose, or leading the horse up to the object, and allowing him to feel and examine it in his own way.

We must be satisfied with our ability to guard against and overcome these difficulties of fear as we can, or as circumstancEs and opportunity will offer. The great point of success is in guarding the horse from being roused to a great sense of danger from any cause, and gradually, as he will bear, force the mind to an understanding of the innocent character of the object or cause of excitement. Familiarity with any kind of danger blunts the sensibilities, and this should be the object sought, after insuring the greatest possible control over the animal. The better to convey an understanding of my meaning, I will give directions for overcoming fear of the most common objects, usually objectionable to horses, which will indicate the treatment for anything else not specified.

A Robe.

While held under careful restraint, let the robe be brought up gently to the colt's nose. After smelling and feeling of it in his own way until satisfied, rub it gently against the head, neck and body, the way the hair lies, as he will bear. Then stand off a little and throw it across the back, over the neck and head, gradually stepping farther, until you can throw the robe upon him as you please. Repeat the lesson several times.

An Umbrella or Parasol.

While holding the colt by the halter or bridle, as may be necessary, bring the umbrella to his nose gently, rub it against the head, neck and body, as he will bear, spreading it a little, repeating the process of rubbing, and so continue gaining little by little, until you can raise the umbrella over the head, and pass it around the animal as you please, without exciting fear or resistance.

Sound of a Gun.

First, commence by snapping caps a short distance from the horse, gradually, as he will bear, approaching nearer, until you can snap caps while the gun is resting upon the back, over the head, etc. Then put in a little powder, and at each repetition increase the charge until you can fire off a heavy load without exciting fear.

Railroad Cars.

Let the animal see them at rest, then gradually lead or drive him up to them, even to smelling them with his nose. Now, as you have an opportunity, drive the horse around while they are moving, working up nearer as you can, and at the same time turning him around so that he can see and hear them from different directions. This lesson should be often repeated, being careful not to crowd beyond what the colt will easily bear, until they cease to attract his serious attention.

Objects Exciting Fear While Riding or Driving.

Should the horse show fear of a stone or stump, or anything of the kind, he will naturally stop and stare at the object in an excited manner. Should the cause of fear be great and sudden, he may attempt to turn round and run away. This is to be guarded against, by sitting well forward on the seat, and taking a short hold of the reins, at the same time speaking calmly and encouragingly to the horse. Bear in mind the horse has a great advantage over you, that his excitement is liable to precipitate his whole strength against you at the least sense of freedom, or additional cause of excitement; that once resisting control in this position, he will try to do so again at all hazards, under like circumstances.

Speak encouragingly to the horse, but keep a close watch upon his actions. In a short time the extent of his alarm will not only be perceptibly lessened, but he will become calmer, and almost disregard the object. Then drive nearer as he will bear, exercising the same patience and care. At each effort to get nearer, the horse will become apparently as much frightened as at first. Keep pushing a little at a time in this way, as the horse will bear, until you can drive up to the object, or by it, and you not only leave no bad impression upon the mind, but gradually overcome the disposition to become frightened.

Sometimes a horse will dislike a wheelbarrow, baby wagon, turkeys, etc., but the treatment is the same. When the excitement is not so great as to endanger successful resistance, and the horse is disposed to "play off, or soldier," it may be advisable to apply the whip a little sharply, but this is to be avoided when it is seen the resistance is wholly induced by fear, and the animal is not lazy.

Some horses while driven to carriages, will not bear the noise and excitement of other horses being driven up behind. This is principally on account of the horse's inability to see and understand the cause of the excitement, or it may be owing to the fault of the driver. Some one drives up rapidly behind, perhaps wishes to "go by," to prevent which the colt is hallooed at and whipped up to prevent such a result. This may be repeated a few times, and the consequence is, if a spirited horse, the habit is acquired of rushing ahead to avoid the punishment expected under such circumstances, and very often, too, a horse is forced into this habit by being run into from behind.

Using Blinders.

It must be remembered that the blinders in general use so cover up the eyes as to make it impossible for the horse to see things plainly sidewise, or at all from behind, which tends to increase the fear, as we are convinced, when we see that to overcome the animal's fear of any object, the first and most obvious point is to give him an understanding of its appearance and character. Blinders are admissible only when there is a desire to conceal the defects of a large head, and to cause a naturally lazy horse to drive steadily, by preventing him from seeing when the whip is about to be applied.

Must See the Object from Different Positions.

It is one of the peculiarities of the horse to understand and be reconciled to an object or cause of excitement only from its position and circumstances as brought to his notice. This seems to be on account of the horse's reasoning powers being so limited as to be unable to retain the same understanding of the object beyond the position from which it is brought to notice.

Every progressive change of position requires almost the same care and patience as that preceding. For example, if in teaching a horse to submit to an umbrella, if it were shown only from the near side, upon carrying it to the off side, would inspire nearly as much fear as at first from the near side, or there may be an aversion to some particular object, or resistance may be inspired only under certain circumstances. You may succeed in getting a colt gentle to be rode from the near side, but an attempt to mount him from the off side, would in all probability be resisted.

If a horse is afraid of an umbrella while in harness, he may be taught to care nothing about it out of harness, but if not taught to feel and understand its character in harness, would be apt to be as much frightened at it in that position, as if he knew nothing about it.

This seems to puzzle many well-meaning men, and is often the cause of much disappointment.

A horse that is afraid of an umbrella, is brought forward to illustrate the management of such habits. In a short time the horse will bear the umbrella over and around him in any manner, without seeming to care anything about it. The owner is pleased with the belief that his horse is broken, when in harness at some future time, he raises an umbrella behind the animal, and is astonished to find him almost as bad as ever, and he naturally condemns the instructions as of no account; and indeed this would seem to be correct. But when it is seen in the first place that it is often necessary to repeat the treatment, that expecting the animal to be broken of the habit by a single indirect lesson, only tends to defeat success. For without ability to control the horse, every attempt to force upon him the object of aversion only inspires greater resistance, because taught to a still greater degree to resist control, and a sense of freedom always tends to increase the animal's fear of the object. Now the efforts of the owner to control the horse directly in a position of so great disadvantage, may produce exactly this result, and then from an ignorance of the cause of failure, believes it is impossible to make the horse gentle.

The lesson must be repeated as long as may be necessary to the end of perfect success, or the horse once excited is liable to drift back to being almost as bad as at first.

Special Remarks on Subjection.

It must be borne in mind that horses of courage and spirit will resist any attempts to overcome their resistance, with the greatest persistency.

If there is great strength and bottom, and the color gray or sorrel, you may look for a horse that will resist you at every point. If the eyes are small and set well into the head, or if the eye-brows are heavy and the expression of the eyes stolid and reckless like those of a mule, you will find pluck of the most determined type. In the management of such, push them as rapidly as you can, subjecting to the first and second methods of subjection as may be found necessary. If the animal is warmed up very much, your difficulty will be increased; and if very reckless, hold your point as well as you can until the system becomes cooled, when the treatment is to be continued, doing so much as the animal will bear until successful.

It is always necessary to success to encourage obedience by the greatest kindness. Indeed, the most severe abuse will be forgotten if as soon as there is submission the animal be caressed and given sugar and salt, apples, or anything of which it is fond. In reforming character, the mind must be toned down by careful, gentle treatment, after the animal yields to the subjective course.

As I have illustrated to you before the class, it is rarely ecessary to resort to extreme measures, as my simple treat ment is so effective as to enable the successful submission of even horses of a very bad character at most in an hour's time. Remember, too, that by the almost absolute control given by my system, you could easily, if imprudent, do harm. I have not only before the class, but in other portions of this book, tried to impress upon the mind the bad consequences of thoughtless force.

If an ignorant, coarse-tempered man were to be given the use of a finely constructed but powerful machine, how soon might he get it out of order and injure it for want of a little patience and care in attending it! Want of oil would in a short time, perhaps, cause it to run hard, and if forced without looking to the direct cause, would only produce greater injury. A little oil in one place, a little readjustment where needed in another, would repair a derangement which perhaps violent force would only increase to an irreparable degree.

While the subjection of horses requires resources of power, the finer faculties of the mind must be brought into play, in determining just where and to what extent this power is to be directed; and remember, the greater your prudence and skill in doing this, the less appearance of violence.

The great point in reforming a horse is to change his character, without BREAKING HIS SPIRIT or in any way INJURING HIM. Now my system of subjection will enable all this, if ordinary prudence is used in its application. I would earnestly urge upon the reader to keep in mind the fact that it is to the strategy based upon the exercise of reason that gives man his position of supremacy, and that to be a really good horseman requires its exercise in directing the efforts in the performance of this duty.

Safety Shafts.

Get three scantlings or poles of good tough timber of about four inches in diameter and fourteen feet in length each. Put down two of these, so as to bring them two feet apart at one end and thirteen at the other. Now lay the other pole across on the ends of the others widest apart, about six inches from the ends. Mark and halve them together. Then bore a hole through both pieces at each corner so fitted, and bolt them firmly together. To fix the other ends, get a piece of tire iron four feet long, and bend it in the form of a breast collar, the rounding side in, so as to have each end extend back on the inside of the holes ten or twelve inches, and fit up nicely to the wood; have two holes punched or drilled through each end of the iron, by which to bolt it firmly to the poles. Then drive staples into or near the ends.

To finish the other ends, take two pieces of iron about a foot each in length and an inch in diameter, flat one end and punch through two holes. Work down the other ends to a sharp point; bend down the ends so sharpened about six inches, in the form of a half circle; bolt these irons under the ends of the poles, the sharp ends pointing down and back, forming dogs, something like those on the ends of sleigh runners, to prevent the sleigh running back. Now harness your horse into this arrangement, taking the precaution to wind the irons across the ends with an old piece of cloth, and strengthening the harness if at all likely to break, by tying a piece of rope around with a piece of breeching, and around the body as may be thought necessary. Though perhaps the best way to hold the shafts, as we call them, nicely up to the neck, is by bringing a strong rope or strap over the neck, and fastening around the iron near the wood. This is a very good means by which to drive unmanageable horses towards such causes of fear as cars, etc. Hitch the horse into the shafts, let the reins run back through the lugs; get behind and drive around, touching up with the whip as may be necessary. If the horse is valuable, and it is desired to take unusual precaution in overcoming fear of cars, or any other greatly exciting cause to drive up to or by, the shafts are good. It is impossible for the horse to run back or sidewise, or rear over back. The horse is almost helpless, so far as being able to run back or sidewise.

Running Away.

This habit may be induced by a great variety of causes—principally by becoming frightened in some way, though often by the horse learning to pull against the bit so hard as to defy control, and is therefore at the least cause of irritation disposed to pull ahead and run away. When actuated by fear, the resistance is usually so sudden and violent as to induce a degree of resistance to the restraint of the bit we have not power to prevent or control. Sometimes, too, the horse will spring sidewise, or turn around in doing this, and will so learn the trick that at the least excitement he will spring into a sharp run. All this resistance, it is seen, results from defective training of the mouth, and is virtually surmounted when able to force so great a degree of control by the bit as to break up all disposition to resist restraint when excited.

Running away is a very serious and dangerous habit, and all such predispositions should be thoroughly broken up when manifested. If very bad, tone down resistance by subjecting the animal to a course of subjection; after which put on the breaking bit and force the most thorough submission to the slightest restraint of the reins.

Let this be very thoroughly done. Then hitch to wagon, making the horse stop whenever called upon or pulled upon by the reins, until there is no disposition to resist, though subjected to the greatest excitement. Some horses subject to this habit will yield readily to the use of the four ring bit. The foot-strap is also a valuable auxiliary, but the breaking bit is in advance of anything else in overcoming this habit. Horses of this character should be made thoroughly manageable before being trusted.

Turning Around.

If the horse turns around, drive first with harness, whip up sharply, then make him stop, always pulling in the opposite direction from that the horse usually turns, until there is not only the most prompt obedience to the commands in going ahead, but ready submission to control, right or left, or in stopping, as may be required. Sometimes the habit is contracted of pulling so hard on the bit as to resist control. In this case all that is necessary to do is to train the mouth once or twice with breaking bit, or use the four ring bit, and the habit will be broken up. If one rein is *pulled upon*, pull sharply on the opposite rein, and repeating at each indication of such a purpose until the head is yielded freely and evenly.

In reviewing the common causes of this habit, we see that two objects must govern the efforts. First: To overcome or neutralize the exciting cause of resistance—usually some cause of fear. Second: To make the mouth perfectly submissive to the most delicate restraint of the bit; it being essential that the exciting cause should be removed, while the power to control resistance must be increased.

I will in this connection add, that there is no part of the training of horses which should be done more thoroughly, or tested more carefully, than this of teaching a proper submission of the mouth to the bit. Yet I will venture to assert none is more imperfectly or ignorantly attempted; and that the more experienced and intelligent horsemen should regard doing this difficult, when there is so much to indicate to the most ordinary observer the method of doing it with ease and certainty, seems strange. And yet, perhaps, this is not so strange, since it has been very much of a puzzle to do this at all, and really in its true aspect shows more real science than can be illustrated in any other feature of my treatment, since upon this must depend ultimately the readiness and success with which the horse can be guided and controlled in harness.

It is essential in training a horse well to the bit, that the idea is given correctly of submitting the head up and back when pulled upon. Also, that the horse should be made to understand exactly the meaning of every signal of guidance and restraint. In training the mouth, the exact idea can be conveyed by being particular in repeating the same kind of reproof, by pulling sharply whenever there is an attempt at pulling hard. There is soon not only prompt obedience to restraint of the bit, but there is no disposition or confidence to resist control. Remember a horse cannot understand the object of such restraint, if there is not uniformity of action and language. Yet most people talk to their horses in the most careless manner. If there is an intention of approaching a horse, the usual word is "whoa!" In driving, when it is desired to make the horse go slow, "whoa" is the usual word, and the consequence is the animal does not know what is meant by "whoa." Every action and word should have a special meaning, and they should never conflict, that the understanding may not be confused. "Whoa" should be an imperative command to stop. To go slower requires the use of some other word. Even every motion of the whip should have a special meaning. If the horse is managed with care in this way, he becomes almost a machine, that yields submission to the slightest touch or word of command.

Running Back.

To break up this habit, there must be established a thorough fear of the whip, so as to induce going ahead when commanded. Put on harness, and tie the tugs into the rings of the breeching rather short. Drive around with the reins, giving a short cut with a good bow whip around the legs once in a while, if not prompt. As the horse learns to spring ahead when commanded, pull a little on the lines, gradually repeating until he will pull quite hard on the bit to go ahead. Make this as thorough as possible. In driving, repeat and carry out this, going ahead promptly, whipping up sharply once in a while if necessary.

The main point to make with horses of this character, is to create a thorough fear of the whip. To do this well while driving with harness, whip around the hind legs sharply, until the horse will start ahead promptly when commanded. Now, attach to wagon, and gradually work up with whip until there is prompt obedience. The foot strap may be put on if there is any possible danger of the horse running back when hitched. A much surer, though more complicated way, is to use the safety shafts.

Kicking in Harness.

This is apparently the most dangerous and difficult habit to overcome, to which horses are subject; yet it is a habit that yields readily to my treatment, but requires care and thoroughness and a large share of common sense in determining how much must be done and when to stop. This cannot be learned by any fixed rule, since there is such a great difference of extremes shown in this habit that it is not safe to venture a limit of what and how much must be done. I have often broken horses of kicking, of apparently the worst character, in twenty or thirty minutes. Then again, one scarcely confirmed in the habit may require very much more time; and a few extreme cases, of apparently a mild character when not excited, would call out all my resources for hours, to make the subject yield safely to control. I broke a horse in Maine of the worst character, of kicking, by a few pulls upon the war bridle. At all events, the owner informed me months afterwards, that the animal remained perfectly docile. This horse would kick at anybody or anything.

But I found a horse in Mississippi, which was perfectly gentle to ride or handle, would only kick when to wagon, yet he was the most terribly persistent kicker when in harness I ever saw, or ever expect to see. All ordinary treatment was only as play to this horse. Circumstances made it necessary to break up the habit, and I felt compelled to do so, and succeeded only after three lessons. Never did a horse resist more bravely, but I succeeded in making the animal so gentle as to submit the wagon against the heels going down hill, and he was driven by me a week after being broken, in the presence of a large concourse of people, proving safe and gentle afterwards.

Breaking of kicking, as with most other habits, requires thoroughness in what is attempted. If there is more fear than willfulness, the fear must be thoroughly overcome. If based upon willfulness, that must be mastered at any hazard.

In either case, put through a careful but thorough course of subjection, exciting resistance by rubbing a stick of some kind against and between the legs until there is no resistance; now put on harness and breaking bit, and compel perfect submission to its restraint. Let the hind legs be touched as before, and at each indication of resistance, punish sharply; with the reins back the animal against a rail fence or anything convenient. If there is perfect submission, back into the shafts of the wagon, or bring the shafts over the back gently. This is a step requiring much caution and firmness. Stand at the left shoulder, grasping the rein near the bit firmly, and as the shafts are brought forward, and the cross-piece comes in contact with the legs, if there is much sensitiveness shown, give him a sharp, quick jerk upon the reins, which will at once disconcert the horse, and at the same time throw the head so high as to make it difficult for him to kick. Force this point well, until the contact of the wagon is borne, when the harness may be attached. Now drive around gently, stopping and starting repeatedly, carefully observing how much forcing the horse will bear. If there is no indication of serious resistance, follow up by driving around, until there is perfect submission. At each repetition of being hitched to a wagon for a few days, let the horse be backed against the cross-piece several times until it is borne without flinching.

This precaution of *testing* repeatedly is absolutely essential to prevent and overcome any growing sensibility or confidence of ability to kick when driven, until there is not discovered any disposition to indulge in the habit.

If this will not do, repeat the lesson of subjection which the reader has been shown, and if there is any doubt about submitting to the shafts without danger of an accident, get two poles about twelve feet each in length; lay them down on the ground so that the small ends will be about twenty-two inches apart, and the large ends are six or seven feet apart. Next get a piece of pole of the same size, lay across and tie firmly to the side poles just far enough from the forward ends so when the horse is hitched in the tugs are tied to this cross-piece with pieces of cord. Hitch to this without hold-backs, and drive around, repeatedly stopping and backing the horse against the cross-piece until there is perfect submission. This driving in poles may be repeated if thought necessary, remembering that it is absolutely necessary to make every step sure before the next is attempted.

A great advantage of repeating the lesson is, that the sensibility of the mouth is so greatly increased that the most plucky horse will scarcely dare resist the bit after being severely punished a few times. If the horse yields, but is doubtful or appears touchy and sensitive once in a while, you may be able to make your point by putting on the foot strap, as directed under that head.

It must be borne in mind that much depends in making subjection thorough, as the peculiarity of treatment is, that no matter how good or proper the treatment, the horse must be made to yield unconditionally, or failure is not only probable but almost certain.

If, however, the horse will not yield to this treatment, it will be necessary to resort to more complicated and slower treatment, by which to counteract resistance, with more severe reproof.

Kicking Straps.

To do this, have made four straps, like common hame straps; two long enough to buckle around the hind legs above the gambrels, and two a little shorter, so as to be in proportion, to buckle around just below the gambrel. The straps should be an inch and a quarter wide, good thick leather, and the buckles should be heavy. Now have made two D's, just twice as long as the straps are wide. This D should have the straight part a little rounding, and the corners not quite to a sharp point. Put a long and short strap on each D, and buckle them around the hind legs of the horse; the long strap above and the short one below the gambrel, bringing the D in front of the leg. These we designate KICKING STRAPS.

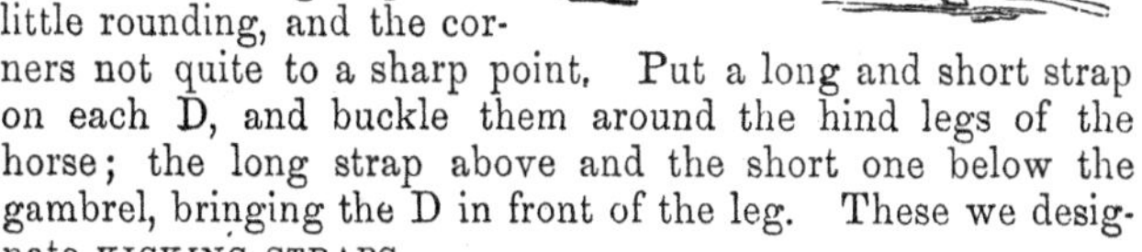

Put a strong well-fitting rope halter on the head, tie a strong two-inch ring on the end of the hitching part, which should be of a length to extend between the fore-legs, over and just back of the belly band. Then take a piece of strong manilla rope, long enough to extend from the ring on the end of the halter back to each hind leg. Pass the end of this through the ring to the center, and tie each end carefully into the D's on the straps, the whole so arranged in length that the horse can travel easily and naturally. Now as soon as the horse kicks, the most severe punishment must result upon the nose. No quarter is to be given until there is perfect submission. The harness may be put on after the horse ceases kicking, and drive around as before. These straps should be kept on until there is no disposition to kick.

If the mouth is hard, use breaking bit and force as before, with the reins, until there is perfect submission. The horse is to be treated with the utmost kindness when he yields. *Bear in mind this rule must not be disregarded*, of addressing and winning the coöperation of the affections as soon as there is submission. The foot strap may be used as a precaution when hitched to wagon, until submission is made sure.

If the mouth is naturally sensitive, and the horse is docile but quick and irritable, a different policy must be adopted, as the horse may drive gently for hours, or even days, and yet may kick at a real or fancied cause of annoyance. This mode of treatment would not work well with such, as they soon become cautious by throwing the head down when there is such an intention, and there is not persistence enough to make reproof sufficiently positive to cure the habit.

The OVERDRAW CHECK will now be just the thing. But care must be taken to apply it right, or there will be cause for disappointment in its use. The object is now to simply disable the horse from his purpose at the least attempt to kick, which we can easily do, especially while in single harness. Probably the best way to do this is as follows:

Get a small steel bit and hang it loosely above the driving bit in the bridle. Put the bridle on the head; now provide yourself with a fine, strong piece of hemp or cotton cord, about three-eighths of an inch in diameter, and sixteen feet in length. Cotton plow line is just the thing, or that kept at hardware stores for hanging windows, will do. Put the center of this cord back of the ears, run the ends back through the rings of the small bit and through the gag runners, which should be close up to the ears. (See cut.) Pass them now through the terrets and back through a ring, which must be attached as far back upon the crouper as possible, and attach the ends to the shafts on each side of the hips. At first this check should be drawn short, to bring the head as high as the horse can bear. The head is now not only high, but the least effort to kick will thwart itself by drawing the check tighter, thereby preventing the horse from doing any mischief. As there is manifested less dispo-

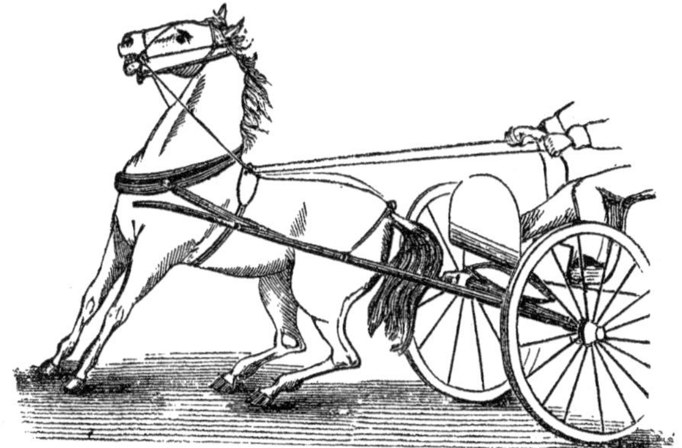

Over draw Check for Kickers.

sition to kick, give more freedom to the head. When the animal proves safe, change and use the common check rein, at first rather short. A nicely rounded strap may be used instead of the cord. I would here add, that I am aware very many will fail to break up the habit of kicking, if the horse is confident and persistent, for want of judgment and firmness. Many of those who use horses, and who think, too, that they are good horsemen, as the term is, are so confoundedly ignorant, rude, and wanting in energy to do anything more than half right, or do more than perhaps half what is necessary, that it is no cause for surprise that they should often fail.

Look first for the cause of resistance, second for the type of disposition, and try to make the treatment such as will prevent and overcome the habit in the most direct and positive manner, always striving to be cool and careful. Treat the horse *kindly, even with marked proofs of affection*, as soon as there is submission.

Kicking while Harnessing.

Put on the war bridle (small loop,) and work up with it sharply right and left a few times, then pull down tight, and tie into a half hitch. While holding the cord in the left hand, step back and pass the hand from the shoulders to the hind parts gently. If this is borne, take the harness in the right hand and work it back gently over the back. As this is borne, untie the cord and tie down, so as to give the mouth a little more freedom. Now go back and handle as before, being careful to be gentle; if there is resistance, punish sharply, tie down short again, and put the harness on. When there is submission, untie, then work back as before; at the least indication of resistance, tremble on the cord until the horse will bear the harness while free from restraint.

Kicking while Grooming.

Some horses are so thin skinned that they can scarcely bear a currycomb on the flanks or legs, and when excited by rough treatment and too severe use of the currycomb, are easily made vicious to handle or groom. Put on the war bridle, and after working up with it, hold tightly, and with the left hand use the currycomb on the back, gradually working to the sensitive part; as there is submission, give a little more freedom to the mouth, and work back lightly. If the horse seems unable to bear the currycomb, use the brush instead, and that, if necessary, lightly. Work lightly and indirectly to the sensitive part, at the same time speaking gently. It is almost impossible to overcome this habit if there is not gentleness and kind treatment.

The currycomb is used too much by most grooms. A sharp toothed, brass currycomb, *must not be used* on a thin skinned horse; use a brush. I should *want* a horse to kick a man out of the stall who would use a currycomb with needless severity, or be otherwise needlessly harsh.

Kicking while Shoeing.

Some horses have a peculiar aversion to having their feet handled, and if once aroused to resistance, from any cause, are apt to become pretty determined in their habit. If the foot is pulled away when taken up, or the horse is excited and injured in some way while the foot is held, the fear of injury is produced and associated with the requirement, which, by the usual pulling, hauling and kicking practices of the shop, makes the horse worse. The least appearance of ability to resist, after being taken in hand, always inspires the horse to renewed confidence and resistance, and if there is not ability or perseverance enough to enforce perfect submission, after trying to do so, the horse is only made more determined in the habit. As the object is to break up the habit, the energies must be concentrated as directly and forcibly as possible, until the horse is so disconcerted and shaken in the confidence of his powers of resistance as to yield to restraint, and submit the feet as required, when submission must be made permanent by patient, gentle treatment. If only a little irritable and restless at being shod, put on the war bridle, draw tight, and tie in a half hitch. The foot can now be handled. Untie in a few minutes, and let the cord be pulled upon a little when disposed to resist, which will distract the attention and cause submission. If the resistance is determined, take up the fore foot and have it held by an assistant; tie the end of the long web around the hind foot above the fetlock. This done, request the assistant to let go the foot and hold by the head; while standing opposite the shoulder, pull upon the strap until the foot is brought well forward, giving loose the instant there is an effort to jerk or kick. Repeat pulling and letting go, until submitted freely. Now step directly behind and pull back, giving, as before, until submissive; then bring the web over the back around across the breast, pulling short enough to bring the foot well forward; pass the end back under the part over the back, and pull tight.

Let the assistant now grasp the web, holding firmly as ever, with the left hand holding the head by the bridle. This brings the leg forward, where it can be handled at will. If this will not do, tie the end of the web or rope around the neck, near the shoulders, in the form of a running noose; pass the other end back between the fore legs, around the hind leg, below the fetlock and back through the loop, around the neck, drawing it through short enough to bring the foot well forward. Pass the end back under to prevent sliding, and retain in the hand. The horse will now be very likely to struggle to get the foot loose. Should his resistance be so great as to endanger injury, you can give loose on the end of the rope. When the horse ceases trying to get the foot loose, rest the left hand upon the hip, with the right pull upon the foot forward and outward. If there is great resistance, pull around by the head, which will enable you to keep him in such limits as you wish. When the struggle ceases, go back and handle as before. When the foot is submitted to the hand, while held to the restraint of the rope, put the cord well back upon the neck, draw it down tightly, and tie it into a half hitch. Then pull upon the foot with the hand as before. If not resisted, untie the strap and take the foot in hand gently. Put it down and take it up, rubbing and handling until there is entire submission. Then carry it back with the right hand, keeping well forward out of danger, by resting the left hand upon the hip, and pulling and yielding to the foot until manageable. Now pass the left hand down the inside of the leg, take it from the right and carry it back gently; put it down and take it up once or twice. Hammer upon it lightly, gradually increasing, until the foot is submitted as required. Now untie the cord and tie it a little longer; go back and handle the foot as before. If submitted, untie the cord, holding the end in the left hand, and handle as before. If there is an intimation of resistance, tremble on the cord, which will keep attention on the mouth, and remind of the previous control until the foot is submitted without restraint. Manage the other hind foot in the same manner, if necessary. The feet of such horses should be taken up and pounded upon repeatedly in the stable, until submission becomes habitual. It must be borne in mind that the smith shop is no place to more than prevent resistance while shoeing, and it must be expected that a very bad horse of this character will not be made more than temporarily submissive by the treatment usually necessary to enable handling the feet to be shod. Indeed, such efforts are well calculated to excite aversion to a shop and being shod, and hence a horse of courage and sensibility is liable to be confirmed in the resistance by such temporary treatment.

Let the horse be handled thoroughly at home, and if necessary put through a course of subjection, handling the feet repeatedly until perfectly gentle. When taken to the shop, if necessary, simply remind that submission must be yielded, and treat gently—caressing and rubbing head and neck the way the hair lies. Colts should not be taken to a shop to be shod uniil thoroughly accustomed to have the feet handled.

Balking.

This habit is usually caused by confusing and overloading, or trying to force too much by whipping when exhausted, or when the draught from some cause becomes too great for the horse to manage, thereby exciting and discouraging the horse before able to settle down to a steady, determined pull. When a horse, and especially a young one, becomes mad, and will not pull when commanded, there should not be a word or an action that would betray an understanding of the resistance. Change position—take up time in some way by fixing the harness or walking around, whistling or singing, if in the mood. There must not be any appearance of anger. Give the horse time to get over the irritation and become willing to use his strength against the collar. Any characteristic of willfulness denotes spirit and sensibility, consequently not disposed to submit to being rudely and injudiciously forced in harness. If double, get both horses to start evenly. This can be done best, and greatly lessen the weight of the load in starting, by standing directly in front of both horses, catching the bits with the hands. Now move the horses gently to the right or left, until the wheel almost strikes the side of the wagon—giving them time to become steady. When you see they are ready, speak with cheerful, encouraging voice, "come boys." If this precaution is taken, there will be no further trouble; but bear in mind that the horses must not now be permitted to go to the limit of their strength. While they are still pulling with energy, at the first favorable place stop them. After ample time to recuperate, speak to them gently to go. It seems to be natural for a horse to go ahead and draw all he can, and it is only when confused, excited and abused in the most unreasonable and imprudent manner, that the disposition is excited to balk. When once the habit is acquired, it is liable at any moment to be persisted in if excited or much force is used.

If there is any treatment to which horses are subject in educating to harness that is unreasonable and needlessly harsh, and should be corrected, it is that of pounding or whipping to make them go, when perhaps the animals are confused and discouraged, and not in a condition to make much of an effort.

The first and most fatal cause of this perplexing habit is the common practice of harnessing horses and attempting to drive them, and make them draw heavy loads, before the mouth is even trained to submit to the guidance or restraint of the bit. I get out of all patience with men who say they are good horsemen, pride themselves for perhaps owning many horses, and always having more or less to do with them, who talk and act as if all that is necessary to do is to "whip the animal through" at all hazards. If this would make the horse go when commenced, it would be pardonable; but it is well known, or ought to be, that whipping in harness, if there is not certainty in forcing obedience, is just what should not be done. The palliative treatment of patience and means of encouragement, if there is not a knowledge of proper treatment, should always be adopted. It is only reasonable that the horse should resist and become fixed in the habit when needlessly excited and abused.

The whip is too irritating, without giving sufficient power to force obedience, and as the will is stimulated to increased positiveness and sensibility it becomes blunted in proportion to the degree the blood is warmed, this advantage of force by the whip decreases, while the resistance is increased, and hence is often a direct cause of failure.

If the whip is to be depended upon, the horse should be driven around in harness, when it should be made to crack keenly around the hind legs the instant after "get up" is spoken, until the horse learns to spring ahead when commanded. When there is perfect obedience, attach to the wagon and move gently, stopping and starting often, until obedience becomes habitual. To prevent this habit the colt should be driven around in harness, touching up with the whip, until the idea of starting at the touch of the whip, and guiding and submitting to the bit becomes prompt and habitual. Then drive slowly and gently for some time after being attached to the wagon.

If the habit is formed, and especially in single harness, it is usually more from resistance to the bit than collar, and if the horse is young he will yield readily to simple treatment. Put through a careful but thorough course of subjection. Then put on harness and breaking bit. Drive around, whipping sharply the instant the horse does not start when commanded, guiding right and left, and stopping at the control of the bit. If there is a habit of LUNGING AHEAD, regardless of the bit, or of not standing as desired when hitched, be positive and thorough in requiring instant obedience to the command *whoa*. Drive around until there is perfect obedience. Then hitch to wagon, gently start and stop the horse repeatedly, gradually becoming positive and commanding in action, until the obedience is made certain. The lesson of driving to harness should be repeated, if there is any disposition to resist. But if the resistance is so positive that this treatment will not do, try the war bridle, pulling right and left, until the horse yields promptly to the least restraint upon the head. There must be kindness and flattery for every act of obedience, and the most positive reproof at each effort of resistance. But too much regard cannot be paid to the value of affectionate treatment when there is obedience. Talk kindly, give apples, oats, or anything the horse likes.

Effect of Kindness.

The impression of kind treatment, gradually showing and encouraging the animal to yield obedience, is certainly very effective, when carried out well in practice. During my early experience I traded horses very often. In this way I became the owner of a pony mare, eight years old. She proved balky, and on inquiry I learned that she had been traded round for years, and had been owned by nearly all the sharp jockeys in the country, being entirely unmanageable. She would neither go down hill or move on a level in harness. Neighbors advised me to prosecute for being imposed upon with such a good-for-nothing animal. Making it a rule not to find fault if cheated, I declared myself satisfied, and concluded to try what I could do with her. I first filled my pockets with apples, led the mare to a secluded piece of smooth, slightly descending road, hauling the buggy by hand; hitched her to the buggy, but did not urge her to go; read a paper the better to show indifference.

After a while she started on a run. To try to make her go slow by pulling, would be equivalent to making her stop, and so let her go until she wore off the sharp edge of her ambition. I now gradually pulled her back, as I could see she would bear, when I reached a descending piece of ground, made her stop, got out of the wagon, talked gently, gave her an apple, then moved forward a little, saying "come Jennie," (her name,) gave her another apple, rubbing her head, as before, and so repeated, for about half an hour. Then would get into the bnggy and make her start; after going a few feet or rods making her stop, but always getting out and rewarding her with an apple. The result was, that Jennie soon not only would start and stop when commanded, but became anxious to obey me. Drove her home; treated her with the utmost kindness; next day hitched her up gently; made her start and stop a few times before getting into the buggy; got into the buggy; soon made her stop, but rewarded her as before. The result was that I soon could depend upon her starting and stopping when commanded. Of course I carried this treatment from a descending to an ascending grade, teaching the mare gradually to use her strength. The result was that she became one of the most willing and pleasant little working animals I ever owned. Sold her in a few weeks. She became the property of a rough, bad man to horses, who, by needless abuse, made her balk on his way home, and she became spoiled. This mare was of a sanguine nervous temperament, naturally willing to do all she could when shown and treated kindly, but would not bear whipping and abuse. Her will was so strong that she would stand bravely, regardless of the most severe whipping. I struck her with the whip but once, when she threw herself down in the harness. There cannot be too much care and patience with young horses that are learning to drive. If a little stubborn, putting through a short course of subjection and teaching to move forward, as before explained, will soon produce perfect submission. If, however, the habit is thoroughly formed, it must be counteracted by direct means. To do this best, hitch the balker by the side of a gentle horse. Attach a strong piece of cord in the form of a crouper, under the tail of the balker, bring forward through the terret and tie to the hame ring of the gentle horse, just short enough to give freedom so long as the horses are even, but the instant there is a disposition to refuse, the whole power of the gentle horse is brought to bear upon the tail, which will cause the horse to jump forward instantly. Stop and start repeatedly, until there is no disposition to refuse moving forward when commanded. Should pulling on the tail irritate and cause kicking, at once remove the cord; tie the end of the hair into a knot; tie the cord to the hair by this knot; bring forward between the legs and attach the cord to the hame ring or collar of the gentle horse, as before. The restraint is now on the tail lengthwise, which has a remarkably disconcerting influence, with great power to force the horse forward when the gentle horse starts. If this should fail, there is but one resource left, which I can here describe, but which is very effective and valuable if properly applied.

Put the war bridle on; bring the part over the neck forward to the ears; now jerk sidewise and ahead, and finally ahead as there is submission, until there is prompt obedience in coming ahead when pulled upon. Hitch to wagon by the side of a true horse. Have prepared a smooth stiff pole about the length of the wagon tongue. Bore a hole a few inches from the large end, and about a foot or more forward of the head bore another. Lay this pole over that of the wagon, the end over that of the true horse's whiffletree, and tie firmly on top with a piece of cord. Now step forward and

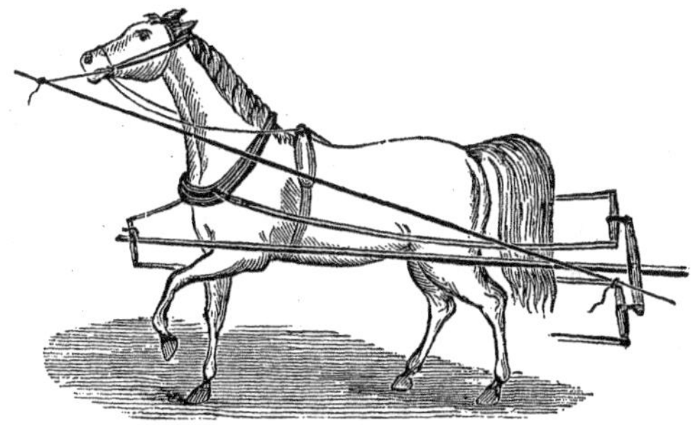

Pole applied for Balkers.

tie a piece of small rope from one hame ring to the other of the horses, under the pole, so as to be just taut when in position. Pass another piece of the same sized cord around the pole and tie it into the true horse's hame ring short enough to hold the pole in the center. Tie the cord on the head now to the pole through the hole, just long enough to give freedom, so long as the horses keep even; but as soon as there is refusal to go, the strength of the true horse is brought by the pole on the head, which will compel going ahead, (see cut.) Start and stop the horses often, until obedience is secured. This pole may be used so long as there is any disposition to balk.

The horse should not be required at first to use much strength in drawing. Let this be required gradually, as there is obedience and willingness inspired to work. It is a grave fault to try to make the horse work immediately. This must not be attempted. First, create a willingness to start when commanded, then gradually increase the load until it becomes habitual to draw when commanded. I am aware very many will have much trouble, and may wholly fail with horses of this character. It is presumed that there is tact and intelligence enough to appreciate and understand the necessity of being patient, prudent and thorough in adapting the efforts skillfully. Those who will not have or have not mind enough to feel the responsibility and value of being governed by reason in the treatment of habits, not only of this type but of any other, must expect a possibility of failure with some very bad horses.

A very good way to work a single balker is to drive first by the side of a gentle horse with the pole, then hitch to single wagon, using two small poles instead of reins to the bit. Now, if the horse does not move promptly when commanded, a little push on the poles will cause him to start, and soon cause prompt obedience. But I would remind again that patience, delicacy and skill in carrying out the principles taught, are the primary and grand essentials to insure success. I would therefore remind, that to illustrate the full value of my theory, it is indispensable that all the firmness, skill and patience possible should be used in directing and controlling the efforts, since without a judicious application of the efforts the advantages may be so far neutralized as to prevent or greatly diminish success.

Kicking in the Stall.

This is one of those habits that require great caution, judgment and care in guarding against danger. Let the horse know by some signal or command, of your presence and intention to approach. Many horses of the gentlest character would kick if approached suddenly and unexpectedly; and again, many horses that are gentle but a little peevish, will not bear being approached without a little care in attracting attention. The motion of the ears and lips, and expression of the eye, will always notify of danger. And here let me warn the reader that however careful he may be in not going too near the horse, there must not be a semblance of fear shown in language or actions. The commands must be low and positive, indicating power. If the horse will not move round and seem to be distracted from a positive intention, stand still, and if the animal does not yield, walk off, carelessly whistling, in such a way that the horse does not see that you feel defeated.

If you have his attention, repeat the words "get around, or over," with a positiveness that must be obeyed, looking at the eye as if you could and would crush all opposition. When you see the horse shrink from your gaze, glide up to the shoulder, before the mind can be made to act, and the next instant let the left hand be passed along the neck and down the head to the nose-piece of the halter, and you are safe, as the horse cannot now kick, strike or bite you. I have repeatedly got to the shoulder of horses in this way that would kick and strike the stall just after I passed, yet not be struck; it is a feat, however, that must not be attempted unless necessary. In going out, the rule is the same—pull the head towards you, looking at the eye sternly; this will throw the quarters from you, and at the instant you let go, glide out and you are safe.

If the horse is dangerous, the safest and best course is to put on the war bridle and make him feel your power by a few sharp jerks of it. Lead the animal into the stall, then step back opposite the hips and say, "get around." If there is not prompt obedience, give a sharp jerk, which will throw the hind part from you. Repeat this, and in a short time the horse will learn to step around promptly when commanded, and allow being approached. If the horse is persistent, leave the cord on, the small loop being left larger and passed above the nose-piece or through the rings of the halter. As you now step out, retain the cord in the hand and hang or tie the end to a nail on the post, leaving sufficient length to permit the horse entire freedom to the halter. Now when you desire to go into the stall, if the horse does not step around when commanded, untie or unhook the end of the cord and give a jerk upon it, which will bring the animal to his senses. Leaving this on a few days, caressing and giving presents of sugar, apples, or anything of which the horse is fond, will soon not only break up the confidence, but so enlist the attention that your approach will be looked for, and eagerly invited to him by stepping around, and endeavoring to reach toward you for the present.

I would here observe that there are very many men who are not fit to have anything to do with a sensitive, well-bred horse. They are either so coarse and harsh as to excite resentment, and hate, or so dull and ignorant that they cannot or will not see that they must both conceal fear and avoid danger. They will not do either. They abuse and show so much fear as both to excite and encourage resistance, and without the genius or tact to correct the cause of mischief they attribute all the trouble to the natural viciousness of the animal.

I would caution also against teasing horses in the stall, or while cleaning, by pinching, pricking or whipping, to "show off," as the term is. Gentlemen who own fine horses should be very particular about this, and a man who would in any way persist in such treatment, or in any manner excite resistance by annoying or abusive treatment, should be at once discharged, whatever his other qualifications.

Pulling on the Halter.

It is the disposition of the horse to persist in what he learns, and this is remarkably so where the habit is one of resistance to the restraint of the halter or bit. If the halter strap is broken once or twice, there is a determined purpose to pull loose at all hazards when hitched. This is sometimes only in the place the habit has been learned. Thus a horse learns to pull loose in the stall—he will resist being hitched in stall, but will submit to be hitched anywhere else; or the horse has learned to pull loose in the street and resists there, but will submit and not pull in the stall. This habit is taught either by being tied by the halter before knowing or being taught to submit to being tied, or accidentally breaking the tying strap. If from the first cause the animal becomes frightened, pulls, and if successful in breaking loose, the habit is established; or the halter strap is so weak that the least jerk upon it causes it to break, the habit becomes fixed.

Put on the war bridle, and train the horse about until he will come to you readily. Now bring the part over the neck forward to the ears, and pull more on a line with the body, repeating until there is prompt obedience to the least pull forward. Wind the cord once around a post, keeping the end in the hand, so as to let it loose a little if necessary. Excite the horse to pull a little, which he will soon fear to do, as there is great pain induced by the purchase of the war bridle in this way. Repeat until he will stand, and let the whip or any other means of excitement be used, without trying to pull.

Should this fail, try the following method:

Get a strong half-inch cord sixteen feet in length; put the center under the tail like a crouper; twist them a few times as you bring them forward over the back; pass forward on

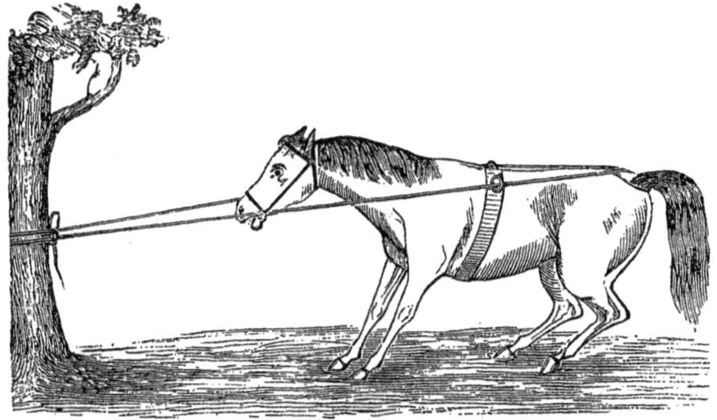

Treating a Halter Puller.

each side of the neck, through the halter ring and tie to the post or manger same as a halter; excite by any means that will make the horse pull until the habit is overcome. To insure safety, would hitch so for a few days, or so long as there is any predisposition to pull on the halter. Same treatment for pulling on the bridle.

Biting and Striking.

There are many habits which to break up successfully require not only good judgment but the highest order of nerve, and this is not only one of that class, but one that requires perseverance and caution. The least want of watchfulness will encourage this propensity; and however thorough the training, if there is not this care, the horse will be encouraged to become aggressive, and once allowed to do so successfully the point gained is lost. Hence the necessity of being able to see the intention at a glance, and disconcert the mind from its purpose before being fully developed. The horse must be made to yield the most perfect submission. If a stallion this is an absolute necessity. If the war bridle will not enable this, put through a course of subjection, and follow up with either the four ring bit or war bridle, punishing sharply. In approaching afterwards, speak sharply "get round!" or any signal that will attract attention. Let the left hand be put on the shoulder, (near side,) glide it up the neck to the head, then down to the nose-piece of the halter. If there is an attempt to bite now, the hand is carried up before the head and held out of reach, while you can keep the head from you with the greatest ease.

An old horse subject to this habit must be watched closely. So long as there is disposition to bite, the horse must not be regarded safe. Carelessness and timidity, especially if subjected to harsh treatment, may be regarded as the primary cause. I have known horses to become inveterate biters by being whipped once or twice.

A gentleman informed me lately that a horse he formerly owned became terribly vicious by being struck once with whip in stall. He was, up to that time, as gentle as any horse could be. One of the most vicious horses I ever handled of this character, was made so by being whipped once severely. He jumped at his owner and would have killed him if not driven off with clubs. He had run in his stall seven months, and would jump at any one with the ferocity of a desperate dog. I made him gentle in less than twenty minutes, and he remained of a good character afterwards. If the horse is young and thoroughly treated, there will be but little trouble in reforming the animal. If old and bad there is no hope of success, unless there is unusual nerve, and genius to make every move just right, and follow up the treatment until the mind relaxes from the purpose, and the affections are won. The habit is clearly a mania when once thoroughly formed.

If the horse is allowed to bite without instant and positive reproof, after training, no matter how thorough the training, the predisposition will be again so strongly developed as to make the animal watch for an opportunity to bite. After forcing obedience, encourage every act of docility. Be continually on the watch for danger and punish energetically for aggression, but immediately encourage obedience by kind, affectionate treatment.

Cribbing.

Cribbing, so far as we are able to learn or judge, is a habit. There may be constitutionally predisposing causes, but it is certain, whatever the pretentions of any one, I have never been given any proof of ability to break up the habit with medicine. Horses will not crib on anything that is lower than the knees. Hence the treatment of tearing away the manger and feeding on the floor, or in a basket. Sometimes sawing between the teeth will stop the habit.

There is but one practical plan of breaking up this habit, and the success of that will depend very much upon the skill displayed in making the adjustment.

The act of cribbing induces considerable contraction of the muscles of the neck, and the larynx is forced down much beyond its natural position. This then is the key through which we must act. Have the throat-latch of the halter hang on a line with the top of the head to the junction of the neck with the head. Take a piece of strap, (good firm leather,) about five inches in length, and as wide as the throat-latch. Drive ten ounce tacks in a row along the center of this strap, three-eighths of an inch apart. File the points sharp and of an equal length. Lay this strap on the inside of the throat-latch where it crosses the larynx, wind a piece of waxed thread around both, at the center and ends of the short strap. Buckle the throat-latch just long enough so that it will not touch the neck when eating or drinking, but will press sharply at the least attempt to crib. The result is that at every attempt to crib the tacks will stick into the neck, which will hurt and disconcert the horse from doing so.

The point of success will really depend upon the perfection and care with which this is kept adjusted. If there is large muscular development on the neck or thick necked, the strap must be buckled shorter than when the neck is well cut out, as it is termed. Make the reproof severe at first. Then keep it so as to touch sharply when a repetition is attempted. If the throat-latch is not on a line with the top of the head, the tacks will rest against and cut the jaw, a little below the junction of the head with the neck. If this is kept on a few days or weeks, and then put on carelessly or taken off, there is likely to be failure; for if the horse finds he can crib once after this is put on without hurting himself, he will try to repeat the effort at all hazards, and will punish himself severely to do so. But if punished at first and this kept where it will sting at the least attempt, it will be likely to cure the habit. It is to be kept on from a few weeks to as many months, according to the age and persistence of the habit.

Getting Cast in Stall.

Drive a staple into a beam, or the floor directly over the horse's head, as he stands in the stall, to which attach a strap or piece of small rope of sufficient length to extend within fifteen inches of the floor. Before retiring for the night, attach the other end of the cord or strap to the top of the halter, making it just long enough to allow the horse to put his nose to the floor. Being now unable to get the top of his head to the floor, he is prevented from rolling.

Putting the Tongue out of the Mouth.

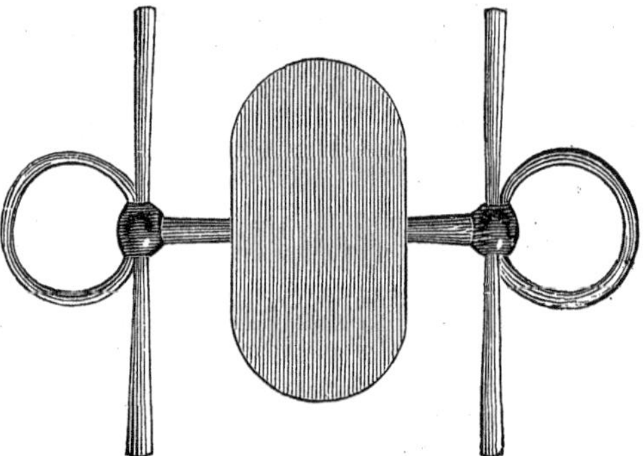

Have fitted a piece of thin sheet iron, about two and a half inches wide, and five inches long, with the ends made rounding, and the edges filed smooth. Drill two small holes about half an inch apart, near each edge at the center. Fasten it through these holes on top of the bit with a piece of small annealed wire. Shorten the cheek pieces of the bridle, so that the bit is drawn well up in the mouth. This piece of iron is now over the tongue, making it impossible for the horse to get the tongue over the bit. Keep this on the bit for two or three weeks, when the horse will become habituated to carrying the tongue under the bit and keeping it in the mouth. The tongue is sometimes, but not often put out under the bit, which indicates a confirmed persistence in the habit, and is sometimes impossible to prevent. The following treatment will work admirably in most cases, and is the only treatment worth explaining:

Get three middling sized bullets and hammer them out to about an inch and a half in length. Drill a little hole through the end of each. Tie one to the center of the bit by a little piece of wire through the joint. Attach the others to the bit about an inch from the center, (one on each side,) so as to play loosely. (See cut.)

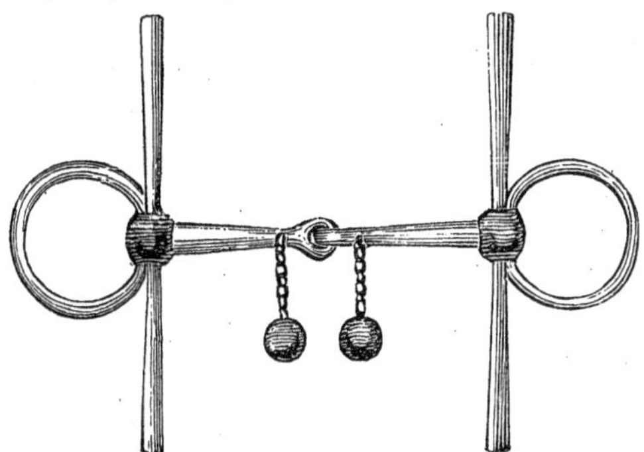

When this bit is now in the mouth, these extra arrangements will so disconcert the horse that in his struggles to get them out of the way, he will forget to put the tongue out.

Jumping Over Fences.

Many farmers assert that this alone is worth the entire expense of the lesson. Certainly if this will prove so valuable, the instruction on Taming and Changing Habits must be invaluable. If a horse or mule, put on a halter that fits well to the head—a five ring halter is best. Next find a piece of thin leather, (an old boot-leg will do,) about as long as the head, and from four to five inches wider than the head is at the eyes. Form it same as cut, with a string attached at each corner. Attach the upper corners by the strings to the halter where the brow-piece is attached to the cheek-piece. Tie the cords attached to the lower corners back of the jaw (being careful to leave just freedom enough to masticate easily.) Let the ends now pass over the throat-latch, and make fast. The horse is simply disabled from looking ahead. He can look

The Jumper.

sidewise and back, but cannot look ahead or over the nose forward, which will disconcert sufficiently to prevent the animal not only jumping, but throwing the fence down. If an ox or cow, attach the upper corners to the horns, and pass the strings around the neck instead of over the throat-latch. I find that cows will not attempt to jump after this has been used two or three weeks. Horses and mules a much longer time, and in some cases must be used for months. Of course farmers should keep fences in good repair to keep stock from being tempted to jump them. It is fallacy to suppose that means, however valuable, can be wholly relied upon for success, so long as the cause is permitted to continue. The leather should be at least four inches wider than the head at the eyes, but five or more will be much better. This will bring the leather outside of the eyes when on, from two to three inches, and around the side of the face to prevent working over the nose. There may be failure with this, but if properly applied exceptions will be rare, as it has proved so far almost infallible.

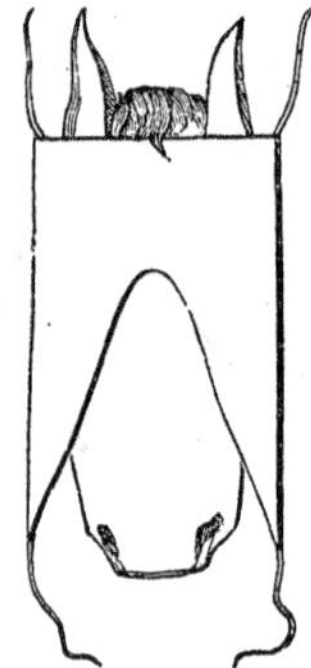

The Jumper.

Pawing in the Stall.

Get a piece of chain about ten inches in length—run a short strap through one of the end links, and buckle it around the foot above the fetlock; or a piece of light chain can be fastened to a small block, and attach it to the foot in the same manner. When the horse attempts to paw, the clog or chain rattles against the foot, and prevents a repetition of the practice.

Kicking the Stall.

The same treatment used for preventing pawing may be used; or a piece of plank may be attached across the stall over the hips about an inch higher than the hips. At each effort to kick now, the hind part will strike this plank and prevent ability to do so. If the kicking is with one foot against side of stall, attach some brush to the side of the stall, or hang down loosely over the part kicked at.

PULLING TOO HARD ON BIT, TURNING AROUND WHILE DRIVING, OR RUNNING BACK, were sufficiently explained in the article on Running Away; which, with the illustration given in teaching, will give sufficient knowledge of the treatment necessary for these and other habits not specially mentioned.

Kicking Cows.

Put on the war bridle, (small loop,) and pull a few times, right and left, then go back gently and attempt to milk. On the least resistance, hold with the bridle and punish sharply, so repeating as may be necessary until the cow learns to stand quietly and becomes afraid to kick. Effectual in every instance.

Of course due attention must be given to the condition of the animal. Sometimes the teats are sore, and the pain caused by milking is very severe. Scolding, kicking, or pounding with the stool should not be permitted, as it only increases the mischief it is desired to avert. One or two lessons have proved effectual in every instance used.

The War Bridle.

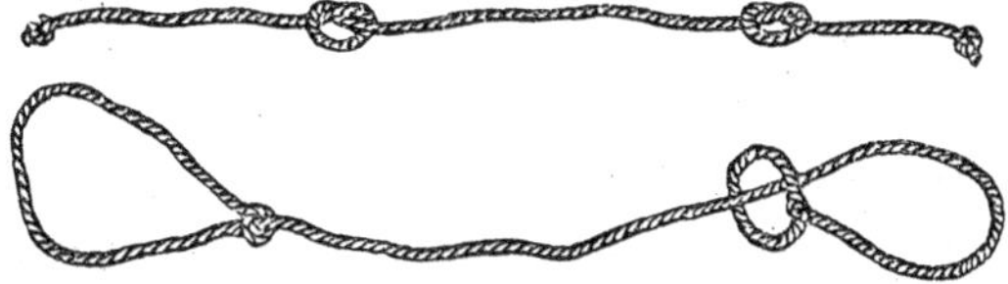

This is simply a fine threaded cotton cord of the best material, twisted hard, of about three-eighths of an inch in diameter, and twelve or fourteen feet long. Tie each end into a hard knot, just as you would do to prevent its raveling, with the difference of putting the end through the tie twice. Then pull down tight and hard close to the end. Now tie another knot about twelve inches from the end, but before drawing it tight, put the end through. (See cut.) This will make a loop that will not slip or draw through. The great simplicity of this form of knot, and the ease with which it can be untied, gives it preference to me over all other forms of knot I have ever used, and is, in my judgment, the best form of knot, all things considered, to be recommended for general use. The peculiar power given to this means of control upon the mouth is liable to cause accident, when used upon a quick, sensitive horse or green colt, with too much energy in such a manner as to bring the restraint directly back upon the mouth, which would in many cases cause the horse to rear up and possibly fall over backward upon the head. Of course a horse is liable to get killed by such an accident, and it must and should be guarded against. This loop should be just large enough to go over the lower jaw, back of the bridle teeth of the horse it is intended to be used upon. The other end can now be formed into another loop in the same manner, with the difference of being large enough to go over the head and fit tightly around the neck near the shoulder.

Applying the War Bridle.

There are two ways of applying and using the war bridle:

1st. While standing forward of the shoulders on the near side of the horse, throw the small loop over the neck and take in the left hand. Then with the right put the large loop through from the top side. Now pass the left hand forward to the mouth, adroitly spreading the loop in the same position over the thumb, second, third and fourth fingers, at the same time the right hand is to be passed under the neck, around the head, upon the nose, which is to be grasped gently but firmly, while the loop is put over the jaw back of the bridle teeth with the left.

By standing near the shoulder and giving a sharp pull, you will find the horse will come to you easily, by repeating which the horse will soon learn to follow. This is a powerful means of controlling by the head; is particularly valuable in teaching to lead, controlling the head, for *forcing*, in bridling, harnessing, grooming, or even in shoeing, if simply a little irritable. Drawing down tightly and tying into a half hitch, will sometimes have a powerful effect. It is not, however, to be regarded as an infallible means, but is a really good, simple means of restraint, and must be used with care. When the horse is of a stubborn, positive character, especially if unbroke, it will be found that there will not always be sufficient power to force obedience with it, though in the majority of cases it will be found to produce very fine results.

2d. Take the large loop between both hands, and while standing directly in front of the horse, slide it over his head well back upon the neck, about where the collar rests. The loop should be made in size to fit tightly around this part of the neck. Now put the other end down between the loop and neck. Put the loop this forms into his mouth back of the bridle teeth, then draw down upon the end until the slack is taken up. This method of using the war bridle, enables more power sidewise than the first, but does not like the first give power to pull ahead.

Four Ring Bit.

This means of controlling the mouth and head gives great power. The knowledge of its use alone, if properly applied, is worth the expense of the lesson and book.

Get a short snaffle bit—steel is best; heat one of the rings and slip over it two inch and a half rings—common malleable rings found in harness shops will do—then bend the ring into form. You have now a common snaffle bit, with two rings on the mouthpiece. (See cut.) Buckle into a common bridle. Get made next two straps, one two feet in length and three-quarters of an inch wide, made like a hame strap; the other about three feet in length, narrower and lighter. Run the short strap through both rings and buckle double, in the form of a nose-piece, buckling just long enough to fit around the nose closely. Bring the long strap around the short one at the center, pass up and through a little loop left in the bridle between the ears and buckle, just short enough to let the nose-piece come straight across the nose. It will now be found by standing in front of the horse, putting both thumbs through the rings and giving a little jerk down and backwards, that the head will be thrown up and back easily. The stop across the nose acting as the fulcrum when the rings on the end of the bit are pulled upon, the two inside rings slide towards the center, forcing the joint upwards against the roof of the mouth, which causes so much pain that the horse will not try to resist after being pulled upon a few times. By tying the end of a small cord around the near ring of the bit, then pass the other end behind the jaw through the

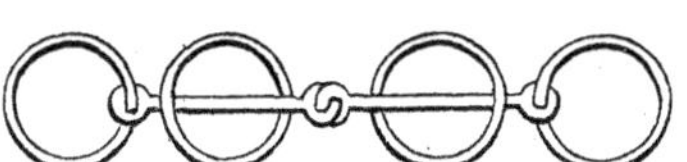

other ring, then over the neck and down between the cord and jaw, (let the part over the neck be set well back,)—now, by pulling sidewise upon the cord, the horse will be found to yield very promptly to its restraint. As a driving bit this is very powerful. After being pulled upon a few times, there are but few horses that will try to resist it. It overcomes pulling on one rein or throwing the nose upon the breast. The effect of this bit on some horses is very great. It does not cut or make the mouth sore like other bits, and would be specially valuable on horses that pull hard and get the mouth sore, as it does not touch the lower jaw, yet forces perfect submission.

Foot Strap.

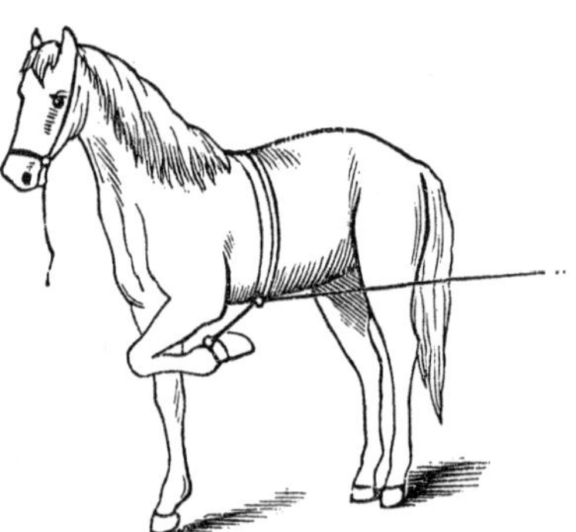

Any piece of strap or rope of about twelve or fourteen feet in length, simply tied around the fore foot in most any manner, will answer on an emergency. But simply tying or knotting around the foot is objectionable on account of the danger of chafing and preventing circulation, or possibly untying at some critical moment. When necessary to use a foot-strap much, it should be specially adapted for the purpose by making as follows: Have a smooth strap made, about twelve inches long and an inch wide, with a buckle on one end and buckle holes punched in the other. About one inch from the buckle should be fitted, under the lap passing around the buckle, a ring or D stitched in nicely. The edges of this strap should be dressed down smooth; or much better, cover the part coming in contact with the foot with a piece of soft leather. This strap is intended to buckle around the foot below the fetlock. Into the ring fasten the end of a strap or web fourteen feet long and an inch and a half wide.

Buckle the short strap around the near fore foot below the etlock, then pass the long strap over the belly-band on the near side back to the wagon, and hold as a rein. This gives control of the foot at will, by which the horse can be disabled and disconcerted instantly, while driving. If the horse attempts to kick, simply pulling the foot up throws him off his balance. He can neither kick or run back, and if he attempts to go ahead it must be on three legs, in a manner that makes resistance quite limited. It is especially valuable when training colts to drive, by neutralizing the animal's power to resist should he become frightened and attempt to kick or back. The foot-strap is also valuable as a means of enabling control of horses that will not submit to being rode, and is very effective.

Trotting.

A good walking gait should be the foundation of the training. Continue this walking lesson until the colt is thoroughly gentle and submissive, and has learned to walk with energy. Now gradually let out on a moderate trot, holding up often, gradually letting out a little faster, as the strength and education will bear, but never so as to cause fatigue. Those muscles that are brought most into use are most largely developed, and bear in mind also that a colt has neither the strength or bottom of an old horse, to bear either much exertion, or to be pushed in his gait, and cannot at once act the part of a fast going, well trained horse.

Let this jogging be continued, gradually as there is ambition and the road is smooth and descending; but let out only so fast, or to the point that the gait is held even and square; and at first should be pushed only a short distance, after which pull back to a walk and speak encouragingly. This is to be repeated, gradually going a little faster, but never to the point of exhaustion, always encouraging with a kind word or two after doing well. I would here caution against hitching the colt to a heavy wagon or sulky. The weight must be reduced as much as possible, and the better to facilitate the object, always let the bursts of speed be on a smooth, slightly descending piece of road. By this precaution you will remove all drag, and the horse is able to use all his powers to the best possible advantage.

This careful driving and gradually teaching the animal to push forward when commanded is to be continued, but however promising, the risk should not be hazarded of trotting a race, or a long distance, before the system is thoroughly matured and hardened to bear prolonged exertion. The gait of many fine trotters is ruined by too much haste and harshness in training. A horse has not his growth until five years old, and should not be put to severe work before six or seven years old. It is proved by experience that much greater age is necessary to attain great speed. Flora Temple made her fastest time of two minutes nineteen and three-quarter seconds, when she was fifteen years old, at Kalamazoo. Dexter is constantly increasing his speed, we are informed, by age and practice; and so it will be found with all the best trotters. They were grown into great speed by careful, persevering work, by which the system is highly developed, the muscles are strengthened and hardened, and useless foul matter that would obstruct the free action of the heart and lungs, and increase the weight, is removed.

Should the horse break when pushed in his gait, he should not be pulled up too suddenly, which would slacken his speed. Rather encourage him to go faster, and by gently and firmly pulling right and left bring him to the trot. The horse has now no disposition to resist control, and he must be taught to rely upon with confidence, as well as yield submission to the control and restraint of the bit.

To Force on the Trot.

There are many promising steppers that will break and run, and will not come down to work again, when much excited; and unless there is power to prevent such a habit and force on the trot, the horse cannot be relied upon in a race, at perhaps the very instant pushing is necessary. There is not power to do this by the bit, and consequently horses that step freely in private become foolish and unreliable when urged in company with other horses. There is but one way of overcoming this trouble, and that is by the use of the following means, the conception of which has been original with myself, and brought to the notice of trainers by me for several years, and has proved in skillful hands a valuable adjunct, to the end of making flighty, nervous horses come down to fast, reliable going.

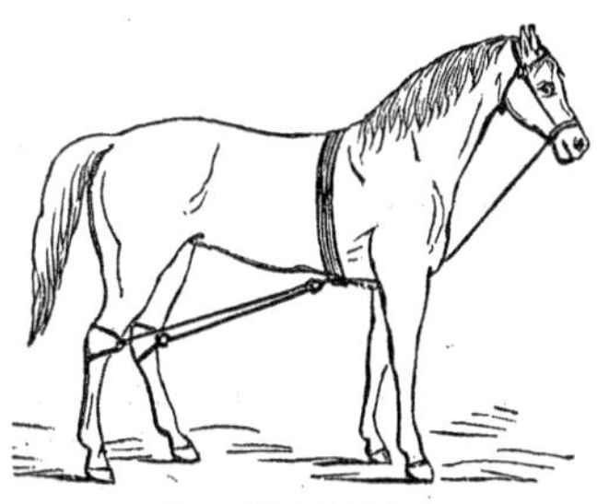
Cure for Breaking.

Have made first four straps long enough to go around the hind legs above the hocks, and from three quarters to an inch wide. Obtain next two D's or rings, in size to admit two each of these straps to be run through. Step in front of each hind leg and buckle these straps around the leg, one above and one below the gambrel, the ring or D in front, bringing the straps to an acute angle. Put on the head a light well-fitting halter. Attach a strap to this, which must be in part double to regulate the angle, and must be long enough to extend from the head to the back edge of the girt. On the end is to be attached a small, nice, easy running pulley, fitted to run a half-inch cord. The strap is to pass back from the halter, between the legs, over the belly-band, just back of which must come this pulley. Take next a piece of firm, hard cotton or hemp cord, from three-eighths to half an inch in size. Run it through the pulley to the center, and tie the ends into the D's or rings attached to the hind legs; the whole to be so regulated in length that the horse can walk or trot easily. This is similar to the kicking straps described on page 45. (See cut.) One leg going forward to the degree that the opposite one goes back, brings no restraint on the cord or head, but the instant both feet go back as in the act of running, the cord is shortened, the head is drawn back, and the horse is taught that he is helpless. He soon learns this and becomes afraid to break, though subjected to any reasonable excitement. With this "rig" on, move the horse on a walk until accustomed to it, which will usually require but a very short time. Then let out on a moderate trot, and when thoroughly accustomed to it pushing to a fast gait. This must be repeated. In fact this arrangement should be kept on until the horse is made reliable. Should be driven and thoroughly practiced with other horses, and excitement made as if in a race. Of course all this requires ingenuity, patience and care.

This will work best on some horses by attaching to the

collar, or around the neck. The restraint is simply more positive by this change.

One gentleman in Ohio, two years since, came one hundred and fifty miles to get this treatment of me, and in three months afterwards he informed me that he had since sold a mare for fifteen hundred dollars which he had bought for three hundred and seventy-five dollars. She would break when in the least excited, and could be made nothing of, though a fast stepper. He bought her, made the experiment, and in less than a month had her down fine, and could hold her under the whip regardless of yelling and the excitement of competing horses. This gentleman informed me he then had a horse that promised equally good results by this treatment.

Breeding.

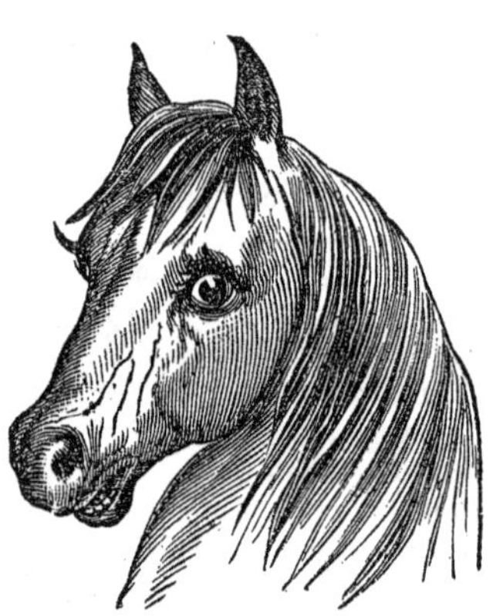

Intelligent and Gentle.

One of the primary points of success is to start right, and in no respect is this more essential than in breeding. The law of like producing like is inexorable; consequently it is seen that to raise good horses, good horses must be bred from. Many farmers who are otherwise keenly alive to their interest, are singularly thoughtless and imprudent in this. If a mare is broken down and unfit for labor, no matter how coarse, badly formed, or what the evidence of constitutional unsoundness, she is reserved to breed from. Again the cheapest horse, no matter how coarse if sleek and fat, is selected and employed to breed from. The most ignorant farmer is particular to select the largest and soundest potatoes, the cleanest wheat and oats, for seed, etc. He has learned this is true economy. Yet there seems to be the most utter disregard of this law of prudence in the breeding of horses and farm stock in general. During my long experience before the public, I have endeavored to impress upon farmers, when I could, that this sort of economy is like paying a quarter for a chicken, and giving a dollar to have it taken home.

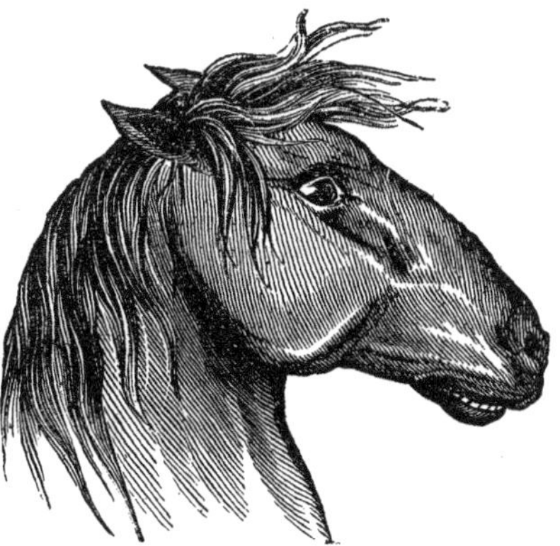
Dull and Treacherous.

It costs just as much to raise a poor, coarse blooded colt, as a fine blooded one. The cost of feeding and care is really the same, the only difference in cost being in that of the use of the horse. The first will possibly sell when five years old and trained to harness, for from a hundred to a hundred and fifty dollars. The other is worth from three hundred to a thousand, and possibly more. The first will scarcely sell for the cost of feeding and care. The second ensures a large profit, and this for a little additional first cost. And then the satisfaction of having fine valuable animals, that can go along if necessary, able to do any kind of work easily, and saleable for a larger price, is a source of no ordinary pleasure and encouragement, if from no other feeling than that of contributing so largely to increased economy and wealth. The fact is, breeding from poor, unsound horses is so much a detriment, that it would be a damage to any one to be compelled to breed from such stock, if given for the purpose. If you wish to raise horses, select good sized, well-formed, sound, fine blooded, good stepping and good colored mares, even though at an extra cost. The stallion

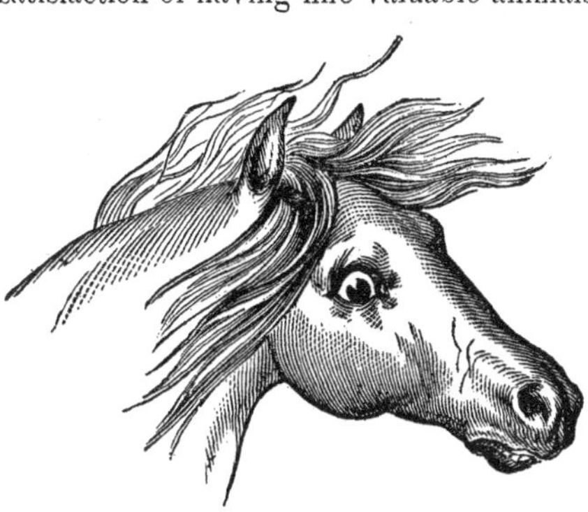
Naturally Sensitive and Shy.

should be free from all taint of hereditary disease. Spavin, ringbone, splints, poll evil, heaves, broken wind, contraction of the feet, weak eyes or blindness, are more or less constitutional; consequently there will be predisposition to such. Strong characteristics and constitutional vigor should be undoubted. This is of course in a general sense.

To be successful in breeding any particular variety of horses requires first decision as to the purpose for which intended. To be particular requires first, intention as to purpose for which intended. If heavy draft horses, evenly trotting roadsters, or ponies are required, select both dam and sire with special reference to the kind of stock wanted. If the mare is light boned or defective, select a heavier boned horse, one that possesses the contrast of greater strength or better points in that respect. But to ensure much certainty of what you would have, the mare and horse should be as nearly the type desired as possible, though not related. I would be very particular about disposition and intelligence. The head should be broad between the eyes, muzzle small, short or middling short from eyes to ears. The smaller and rounder the eyes, the more positive will be the temper. (See cuts.) To have a horse sensitive, intelligent, courageous, and naturally docile, there must be large brain, the eye must be large, standing well out, and mild in expression.

Of course it is understood that BAD TREATMENT WILL SPOIL THE BEST TEMPERED HORSES, AND GOOD TREATMENT WILL MAKE GOOD SAFE ANIMALS OF THE WORST.

The Mare.

The mare is said to go with foal eleven months or three hundred days; but it is not uncommon for mares to have fully developed foals in much less time, and in many instances mares have been known to go four or five weeks beyond this time. Time should be so arranged in putting mares, that the colts will come at a time when there is some grass, as the mare will do better not to be confined to dry feed. The virgin mare, or one that has not had a colt, for one season, must be put when she is found in season. The mare that has had a colt will be found in season, and should be put on the eighth or ninth day after foaling; some prefer the eighth, others the eleventh. Good judges claim that it is dangerous to go beyond the tenth, as the mare is apt to come off her heat soon after, and if allowed to go to a later period, the sucking of the colt is likely to reduce the mare too much to allow conception to take place, and thus a year's service of the breeder is lost.

After putting a mare the days for trial are the ninth after service, the seventh after this, the fifth after this again. Some commence again, commencing with the ninth day and follow up as before, making forty-two days. Twenty-one days being the period elapsing between a mare's going out of heat, and coming in again, making her periodical term thirty days. Twenty-one days is claimed to be sufficient to prove a mare.

After conception, the mare, if allowed to go free, will stand by a fence or tree in a partially dormant position until after the heat passes off. If at this time she is overworked or frightened, she will be likely to cast the conception, and will require to be served again.

After the mare has been a few weeks with foal, moderate work will not only do no injury, but will be of service to her, but at no time when she is with foal must she be placed in a situation where she will be at all likely to receive severe jolts, kicks, or any other violence. Another great preventive to conception, is turning mares out with string proud or badly castrated horses, as they are a cause of positive annoyance to them, and greatly endanger the certainty of conception.

A fine mare was put to a horse, she was proved on the regular trial day, and showed all the signs of conception. Three weeks after being served she stood quietly by a fence, and the owner coming up, thinking her sick, started her suddenly. The fright so shocked her nervous system that she sickened, lay down and cast the embryo. Another in the same neighborhood aborted from a horse teasing her.

A gentleman put a mare that had bred several colts, and after being served to the horse she was allowed to run in a pasture adjoining one in which a string proud horse was kept. She was teased by him, and the consequence was she had no colts for two years. The cause of mischief was finally mistrusted, the mare was put in another field away from the horse, and she did not fail to breed afterwards.

It is a well-known fact also, that if a mare is near food she likes, and is denied being given some of it, there is danger of abortion being produced. I might enumerate a great many cases illustrative of the fact that causes in themselves slight may produce abortion. Much care is necessary. Persons owning mares that have failed to conceive, should be unusnally cautious, as mares having aborted once, are predisposed to do so sometimes from the most trifling causes.

It is a noticeable fact, also, that subjecting the mare to abuse, or great fear from any cause, affects the character of the colt powerfully.

Calling the attention of a class to these causes of mischief, one of the gentlemen corroborated my assertions by making the following statement: He and a neighboring farmer owned two cows. His was extremely wild and intractable; the other was very gentle. The informant said he treated his cow with care and kindness. The man owning the gentle cow was in the habit of making his dog drive her up to milk, the dog causing her to run and be much excited. The cows had fine bull calves. The owner of the wild cow bought the calf of the other, and in time broke them to work, and he said that the barking of a dog or any noise, would make the steer he bought act wild and foolish; that he was naturally wild and untamable, while the other, which he raised himself, from the wildest animal, was as gentle as any steer.

I could refer to many interesting instances of colts showing the marked effects of abuse and excitement on the mother. This is not to be wondered at, since it is seen that the brain controls and regulates the action of the developing brain and nervous system of the fœtus or colt. Such causes should be carefully guarded against.

A stallion of a known vicious character, should not be bred from. The horse should be in vigorous health, and this implies that he has been subjected to moderate but regular exercise, during the season. A horse, however, that is driven and hurried from place to place, over-heated perhaps, and made to cover from three to seven mares, should be regarded as unsafe. They are not sure, and the progeny of such are liable to lack vitality.

After the colt comes, the mare should be allowed to stand idle for three or four weeks, until she gets her milk and has time to regain her strength; and the foal also requires time to acquire strength. It is injurious for the colt to run with the dam on hard roads, to an extent at least that would strain or exhaust. Above all other times in the life of the horse, at this period, and during the first winter, bad treatment is most injurious. The mare and colt should be well fed, and protected from storms. The theory of working a mare hard, and half starving the colt, is the poorest kind of economy, since the mare needs generous feed and rest, to renew her strength and make her milk, by which of course the colt is nourished and made to grow. When size and strength will indicate that it is time to wean, which is usually in five or six months, put the colt in a quiet pasture, away from the mare, where it should be closely looked after. A little oats, (better if bruised,) should be given daily.

The conclusion of careful breeders is, that it is much better for a colt to run in pasture, than to be confined in a stable. If the colt is intended for farm use, castration may be performed when six months old; if, however, the withers are light, it should be postponed until the head and neck fills up to the degree required, and this may require from one to two years, or even more. If the head is large and heavy, early castration is advisable. Colts should be generously fed, and protected from the inclemency of the weather in winter. They should be treated gently. May be broken early to harness, if treated gently and with care. This, however, is hazardous, as there is danger of over-driving young colts if they are driven at all. Many seem to take pride in trials to which they subject two or three years old colts. It is not what they can do, but what they ought to be required to do.

To become well posted on this interesting subject, the reader should get the works of different authors. A little money employed for books on this as well as kindred subjects, will be found to be wisely used, but they should be read carefully. The limit of my space, even if more competent to develop this subject, will not admit of more than a few general remarks.

Feeding.

Hay, corn fodder, oats and corn, constitute the principal food of horses in this country. Hay and oats in the Northern States, fodder and corn in the South. The food should be in quality and quantity to impart strength, vitality and elasticity, and this requires some discrimination and care, as the food should be harmonized both to the condition, and the severity of the labor to which the horse is subjected. As a rule, the stomach should not be distended with food when prolonged, energetic effort is desired, as the heart and lungs would thereby be much impeded in their action, and congestion and rupturing of or enlarging of the air cells of the lungs may result. This is to be especially guarded against in the feeding of hay. Greedy eaters can and will gorge themselves by eating so much hay as to be unfit for active labor, and is usually shown to result in heaves or broken wind. Heaves are always found in the teamsters' or carters' stables, where there is no care in feeding. This disease is always found among horses of the above class, but never found among racing horses, from the fact that the utmost prudence and care is used in selecting the food, and feeding in smaller quantities, or in adapting the food more perfectly to the wants of the system.

It has been demonstrated beyond doubt that the reason horses improve so much in wind by eating prairie hay is, that it is so coarse that horses cannot eat it fast enough to overload the stomach. The quantity of hay should be carefully regulated, and never as much given as the horse will eat if at all voracious. The majority of owners pack a large rack full, allowing either liberty to eat too much, or making it unpalatable and unhealthy, by being breathed upon. From eight to ten pounds is about the average quantity for an ordinary roadster to be allowed in twenty-four hours, more or less, according to size, the kind of work, and the quantity of grain given. Dusty or mouldy hay should not be fed, as it is liable to produce various forms of disease.

All food should be clean, and in quality perfect. Hay is most perfect when it is about a year old. Horses would perhaps prefer earlier, but it is neither so wholesome nor so nutritious, and may purge. When it is a year old it should retain much of its green color and agreeable smell.* The blades of corn pulled and cured in the summer are unquestionably much better than hay. I should certainly prefer this kind of fodder to any kind of hay, for fine horses. It is strange that it is not prized more highly in the North.

Oats make more muscle than corn. Corn makes fat and warmth. Hence, the colder the weather, the more corn may be given, and the harder the work, the more oats. Oats should be a year old, heavy, dry and sweet. New oats will

* NOTE 1.—In packing or stacking hay, salt should be slightly sprinkled through it so as to destroy insects. It also aids in preserving it bright, and makes it more palatable and healthy for the horse.

weigh from ten to fifteen per cent. more than old ones; but the difference is principally water. New oats are said to be more difficult to digest, and when in considerable quantity are apt to cause flatulency and derangement of the stomach and bowels. The same may be said of corn. If not sound and dry, it may be regarded even much more dangerous than oats, and should not be fed. Doing so will be at the hazard of the consequences above mentioned.

The quantity of oats given daily may vary from eight to sixteen quarts. If the horse is large, and the work is severe, a little more may be given. Corn should be fed in the ear, and like oats must be regulated in quantity to the size and labor of the animal; from five to twelve good sized ears are a feed. I give a larger proportion of feed at night, and less in the morning and noon. There is ample time for digestion during the night. There is not during the day, if the labor is severe. Experience proves that some mildly cooling laxative food should be occasionally given. A bran mash, made by pouring boiling water on eight or ten quarts of wheat bran, covered over until cool and fed at night, from once to three times a week, is the finest and best.

Carrots are a good laxative and alterative before frost, but are too cold and constipating during cold weather. They may be fed in October, November and December, but in the Northern States not later. (I am governed by the judgment of one of the best veterinary surgeons in the United States, based upon careful and critical observation of effects on a large number of horses, on this point.) I feed Irish potatoes, from one to three quarts, with the usual quantity of grain, from two to three or four times a week, and would recommend their use. Think their value cannot be over-estimated. Feeding a small quantity of roots and giving bran mashes, keeps the bowels open and the system in a uniform, healthy condition. Without them constipation is probable, and this is one of the primary causes of diarrhœa, colic, or inflammation of the bowels. If it is desired to make a horse fat in a short time, feed corn meal and shorts, with cut straw, to which add a pint of cheap molasses. Nothing like this for recruiting and filling up a horse that is out of sorts or poor. If the horse eats too fast, put a few round stones in the feed box. He must now pick the food from among the stones, and thus he is compelled to eat slowly.

If the horse is exhausted, or when sufficient time cannot be allowed for him to eat and partially digest a full meal, he may be greatly refreshed by a draught of warm gruel, or in summer, of cold water containing a small quantity of meal. To give some idea of the routine of feeding and watering when great care is necessary, I include the system of feeding and watering Mr. Bonner's famous trotting horse, Dexter.

"At six every morning, Dexter has all the water he wants, and two quarts of oats. After eating, he is 'walked' for half an hour or more, then cleaned off, and at nine has two quarts more of oats. If no drive is on the card for afternoon, he is given a half to three-quarters of an hour of gentle exercise. At one o'clock he has oats again, as before, limited to two quarts.

"From three to four, he is driven twelve to fifteen miles; after which he is cleaned off and rubbed thoroughly dry.

"He has a bare swallow of water on returning from the drive, but is allowed free access to his only feed of hay, of which he consumes from five to six pounds.

"If the drive has been a particularly sharp one, he is treated as soon as he gets in, to a quart or two of oat meal gruel; and when thoroughly cooled, has half a pail of water and three quarts of oats, with two quarts of bran moistened with hot water.

"Before any specially hard day's work or trial of his speed, his allowance of water is still more reduced."

Watering.

If a large quantity of cold water is taken into the stomach while the system is agitated and sensitive, by the circulation being so increased as to open the pores of the skin freely, it is liable to so chill the stomach as to derange the circulation and close the pores of the skin, and thus excite some one of the common alimentary derangements of colic or inflammation of the bowels. Hard water, especially cold well water, is more liable to cause mischief in this way than soft water. Hard water will derange some horses, so much as to show an almost immediate effect of causing the hair to look rough or stare, the appetite deranged, if not indeed preceded by colic or inflammation of the bowels; also, horses that are raised and worked in the country, where the water is strongly impregnated with lime, are troubled a good deal with intestinal calculi, *i. e.*, stone in the bladder. Hence soft water should be given, if convenient; and if well water, especially while warm, it should either have the chill taken off or be given very sparingly.

The best time to water is about half an hour before feeding. While driving, the rule should be little and often. None, or only a swallow or two, should be given at the close of a drive, until cool. If very warm, the horse should be walked moderately where there is not a current of air to strike him, from ten to thirty minutes, as may be found necessary. If, then, any danger is apprehended, the chill should be taken off the water if very cold and given sparingly a few swallows at a time. The common custom is to give about a half bucket of water. The safest course would be to give less and repeat. The rule should be, for ordinary use, to give small quantities often during the day, and the animal to pursue his journey or labor immediately after. If allowed to stand, the system may be chilled. The absorbents are closed, which is the common cause of Laminitis or Founder, although this disease may not develop itself until twelve or twenty-four hours afterwards, and any cause which will chill the system—either cold winds or cold water—while the animal is warm, will be almost sure to produce the above disease.

TEACHING TRICKS.

Do not hurry a horse too fast in his training. If you undertake to teach too much, or too fast in the start, or indeed at any time, you only confuse or discourage. Do only so much as the horse can comprehend, and make daily progress.

Teaching to Follow.

If it is desired to simply teach the horse to follow promptly with halter or bridle on, apply the war bridle, (small loop;) when he comes round promptly, stand off a short distance and say, "Come here, sir." If he does not come to you, give a sharp pull, gradually changing positions and going a little farther. If he comes to you promptly, caress him; if not, pull sharply, repeating in this way until you can make him come to you promptly, in any direction, at the word.

To Make Follow with the Whip.

The simplest and easiest way of doing this, is to work up sharply with the war bridle, and when the horse comes to you promptly, take a short, blunt whip, step up to the shoulder, and while holding the bridle loosely in the left hand, pass the whip gently over the shoulder, and tap lightly with the end on the off side of the head. This will annoy the horse and cause him to move the head a little from it, toward you; instantly stop and caress, then repeat the tapping again; should he attempt to run from you, hold him by the bridle. Repeat in this way until the horse will step toward you promptly. Then touch the whip over the hips and say, "Come, sir." If he comes up to you, or shows the least disposition to do so, caress, and so continue until he will come up promptly. Now step a little sidewise and ahead and say,

"Come, sir." If he should step after you, caress, if not, touch the lash over the hips. In a short time the horse will learn to step to you, and follow promptly. When he will do this, stand him in a corner of the room, stand a little in front of him and touch him lightly with the whip on the fore-legs and say, "Come here, sir." At the least intimation of coming, stop and caress. Then repeat, touching with the whip. If he moves to you a little, stop and caress, and in this way repeat until he will come to you promptly. Then get a little farther from him and repeat in the same manner until he will learn to hurry up to you, to get away from the whip. Should he bolt away, put on the bridle, and hold the end in the left hand. You can now hold him by the bridle when he attempts to run, until he finds he cannot get away, and will come up promptly.

This lesson should be made very thorough before there is an attempt to take the horse out of doors, and then in a small yard. If this is not convenient, put on the bridle, having good length of cord, and hold in the left hand loosely.

If the horse is of a bad character, the following method may be used: Turn the horse into a room or small yard well enclosed. Provide yourself with a good bow whip. The horse will feel uneasy and look around at you, and then perhaps for some place by which to escape. Walk up to him, and as he runs into a corner apply the lash sharply under his flanks, following him up, making the whip sting keenly around the hind legs. When he stops or turns his head toward you, stop instantly, reach out the hand, at the same time approaching gently. Should he run or turn around to kick, whip instantly as before, and so continue until you can approach and caress the head and neck a little. Then say, "Come, sir," at the same time touching the whip lightly over the hips. If he comes, or shows the least disposition to do so, caress and speak encouragingly. If he runs, whip as before, and so repeat until the horse will come up promptly when touched by the whip.

As the object is to make the horse honest in following, it is necessary to make him feel that you whip him only for resistance, encouraging and flattering for every intimation of obedience, until he realizes his safety from the whip to be in coming to you.

To Lie Down.

Tie the bridle reins into a knot back of the neck. Throw your strap over the back, under the body, and tie to the near foot, below the fetlock. Now pass the right hand well over the back and take a short hold of the strap. Cause the horse to step toward you and pull the foot up. Then pass the left hand around the reins and pull back and down upon them in such a manner as to turn the head a little to the off-side, at the same time pulling down steadily but firmly on the strap over the back with the right hand. As the horse goes down, gradually pull the near rein, so as to bring the head to the left, at the same time pressing down and from you firmly with the right, until the horse will lie down.* Pass the end of the strap now through the ring of the bit and draw through gently, step over the neck, and as the horse attempts to get up, pull him back, until he lies quiet. Rub and caress him, and after lying a few minutes, say, "Get up, sir." Repeat in this way for a few times until the horse will lie down readily. Then while holding him on or near the knee with the strap, hit him on the shin of the other with a little whip, until he will bring it under and lie down. After awhile he can be made to come on his knees and lie down by simply pulling the head down a little and hitting the shins with the whip, at the same time saying, "Lie down, sir," repeating until the horse will lie down to the motion of the whip. This is about the easiest and most practical way of teaching a horse to lie down.

To Sit Up.

When the horse will lie down promptly, put on him a common collar, and while being down take two pieces of rope, or anything suitable, about ten feet each in length. Tie the ends around the hind feet, carry them forward between the fore legs and bring them once around the collar. Now step on his tail, take the bridle reins in the right hand, while you hold the ends of the ropes firmly in the left. Give a little jerk on the reins and say, "Get up, sir." When the horse throws out the forward feet and springs to raise himself on the hind feet, he finds himself unable to complete the effort, on account of the hind feet being tied forward under him, and so he brings himself in a sitting position. Instantly step forward, holding the ropes firmly, rub and caress the head and neck a little for a few seconds, then as you see the effort to keep up becoming tiresome, let loose and say, "Get up, sir." By repeating in this way a few times the horse will soon learn to sit up when commanded without being tied.

To Make a Bow.

Take a pin in your right hand, between the thumb and fore-finger, stand before, but a little to the left, of your horse, and prick him on the breast lightly. This produces the sensation of a fly biting, to relieve which he will bring down his head, which you will accept as yes, and reward for by caressing and feeding as before. Then repeat, and so continue until he will bring his head down the moment he sees the least motion of the hand toward his breast, or you can substitute some signal which he will understand readily.

To Say No.

Stand near the left shoulder, holding the pin in your hand, with which prick him lightly on the withers, which will cause him to shake his head. You then caress as before, and so repeating, until he will shake his head at the least indication of touching him with the pin; you can train your horse so nicely in this way in a short time as to cause him to shake his head or bow by merely turning the hand a little, or moving it slightly toward him.

To Kiss You.

Teach him first to take a piece of apple out of your hand. Then gradually raise the hand nearer your mouth, at each repetition, until you require him to take it from your mouth, holding it with the hand, telling him at the same time to *kiss you*. He will soon learn to reach his nose up to your mouth; first to get the apple, but finally, because commanded to do so. Simply repeat until the horse understands the trick thoroughly.

Teaching a Horse to Dance.

Put on the war bridle; hold the cord some four or five feet from the horse's head, and with a whalebone whip tap him on the shin or ankle until he lifts his foot, then caress him, and do the same with the other, making him raise first one foot, then the other, then stop and caress. Next, make him raise them several times, until he moves his whole body by the motion of the whip to the time of music. Caress and encourage frequently.

Teaching a Horse to Waltz.

After he has learned to dance, put a surcingle around his chest and fasten the bridle-reins to it, the left rein much the tightest, bringing his head well round to the left side. Then make him move forward, when he follows his head, and every time as he is turning his head from you give him a sharp cut with the whip, which will make him jump round quickly until his head comes around to you again. Then you should caress and encourage him by talking kindly, patting and feeding him. He will then be slower to move his head from you, but you must continue with the whip every time the horse's hind parts are toward you and his head from you, caressing every few minutes until he understands to move at the motion of the whip. Patient and careful practice in this way will make your horse prompt and graceful in his movements.

SHOEING.

THE hoof of the horse, in a state of nature, is adapted only to a grassy surface. Here the natural wear and tear of the hoof is just compensated by its growth. When the wear is made greater than this, by driving on hard roads, the horn is worn down so rapidly that the vascular part of the foot would soon be exposed, and the horse would in consequence become lame. To prevent such a result, much attention has been given to the art of protecting the feet from increased wear and injury.

The first step towards shoeing horses was by fastening a sort of sandal to the foot by means of straps or strings, and as experience brought improvements, plates of metal were used, but fastened to the foot in the same clumsy manner. It is supposed that plates of metal, or shoes, were used and attached to the feet in this way for nearly a thousand years before it was found practicable to fasten them with nails. The first effort to fasten shoes to the feet by nailing was by driving the nails down through the crust and shoe and riveting on the under side. It is not known by whom or exactly when this improvement was made, or when the present system was introduced.

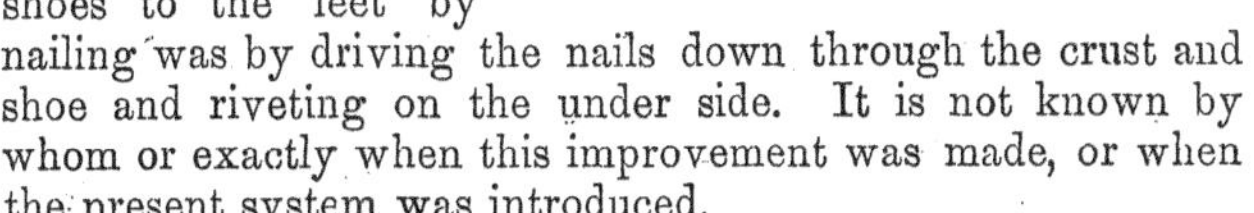

The Icelanders form a piece of ram's horn into shape, and fasten it to the foot by means of horn pins. The antlers of deer are used for the same purpose, according to the accounts of travelers, by people of other remote regions. In Japan sandals of plaited straw are used, fastened with straw bands around the fetlocks. The Arabians use a simple plate of iron, with a hole in the center, nailed on.

Shoeing includes, first, the duty of preparing the feet for the shoes; second, forming the shoes to the feet, so as to be most exact in size, weight and fitting to that part of the hoof, and that only, that is shown by experience to be best able to bear the pressure and strain of the shoe without injury, and preserve its form and bearing best; and, third, that when injury and lameness results, the cause, at least, should be removed, and a reasonable effort made to restore the parts to a state of health.

That part of the foot which is visible, and to which the shoe is fastened, is called the hoof. It is simply a thin covering of horn to the delicate but powerful mechanism of the internal structure of the foot, and for convenience of description is divided into three parts, the wall, sole and frog.

THE FOOT.

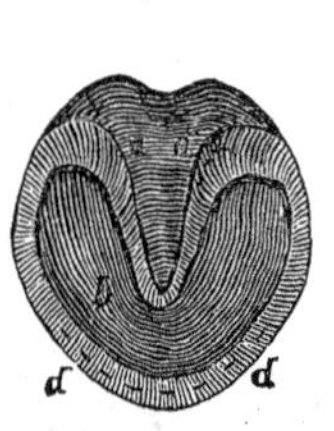

(No. 2.)

a a The frog.
b The sole.
c c The bars.
d d The crust.

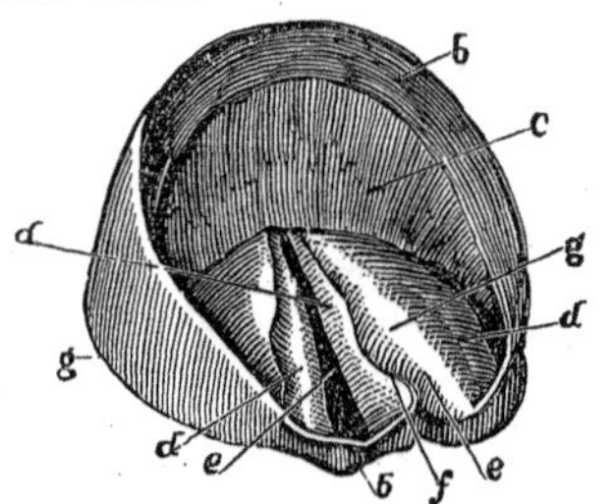

(No. 1.)

a The external crust seen at the quarter. *b* The coronary ring. *c* The little horny plates lining the crust. *d* The same continued over the bars. *e e* The two concave surfaces of the inside of the horny frog. *f* That which externally is the cleft of the frog. *g* The bars. *h* The rounded part of the heels, belonging to the frog.

There are other minor points, a full description of which is not essential to our object here, such as the toe, heels, bars, commissures, &c. The outer crust, or wall, is a simple piece of horn, of from a quarter to three-eighths of an inch in thickness, increasing in thickness from the quarters to the toe, where it is thickest and grows fastest, in order to bear the increased wear upon this part. If this horn were cut into and examined with a microscope, it would be found to be made up of a large number of little tubes, or hairs, cemented together; that they can be split apart like the fibers of wood, and that the horn increases in hardness and density from the inner surface to that of the outer, the inner surface being quite soft, while the outer surface is hard and smooth.

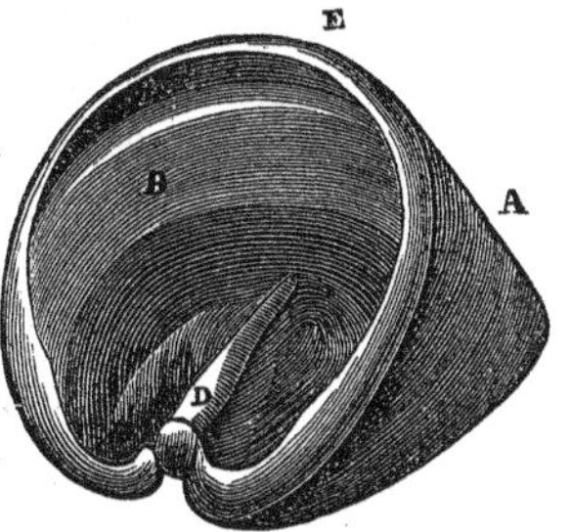

(No. 3.) Interior of a Healthy Foot.

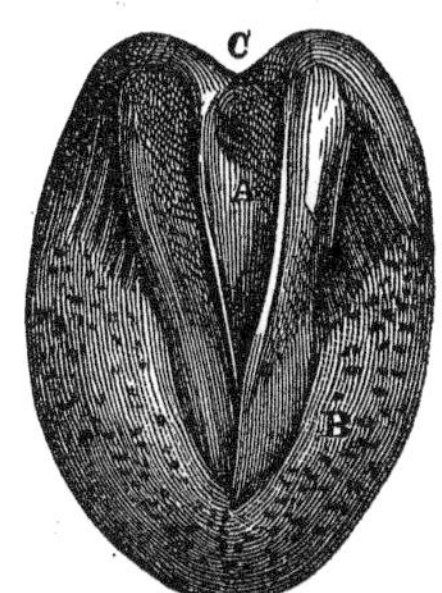

(No. 4.) Sole of a Healthy Foot.

If we now look at the sole, we will find it from one-eighth to three-sixteenths of an inch thick, a little arched, of a dense yielding texture, joined firmly to the lower and inner edge of the wall. At the center, occupying the space between the heels, and extending well forward to a point towards the toe, is a softer and thicker formation of horn, admitting of great elasticity, which is the frog. (See cut No. 2.) Between the frog and its connection with the sole, on each side, is a little strip of hard horn, extending from the heels forward, called bars, which are a continuation of the outer wall. From the outside there seems to be a deep notch, on each side, cut down between the bars and frog, which are called commissures, the whole showing the most admirable arrangement for strength and elasticity. The frog, being of a soft, elastic nature, acts as a cushion in protecting the sensitive parts over it from being bruised or injured, while the direction of the bars make them braces for keeping the heels in place. Connecting the internal parts of the foot with the

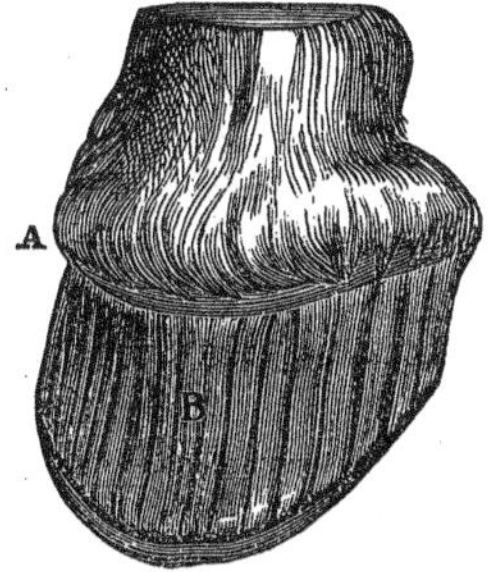

(No. 5.)
a Coronet.
b Sensible lamellae.

hoof, is a strong muscular structure, arranged so as to affo great expansion, as well as strength. That connecting wi the wall of the hoof is named sensible laminæ, and th between the coffin-bone and sole sensible sole and frog. Th muscular structure has mingled through it a complete network of nerves and blood-vessels. Hence we see that in any way producing pressure or restraint upon the wall or sole, so as to bruise this soft structure, will cause inflammation, and result in soreness, change of structure and lameness, to a greater or less extent, in proportion to the extent of the injury.

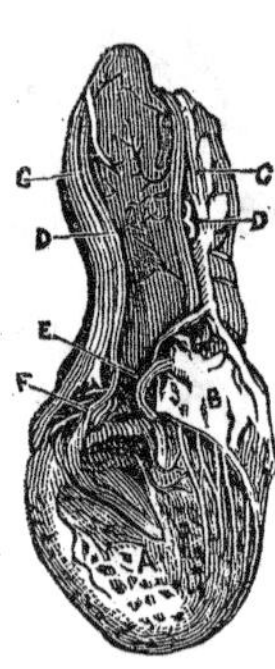

(No. 6.)

View of the Arteries of the Frog and Sole, injected.

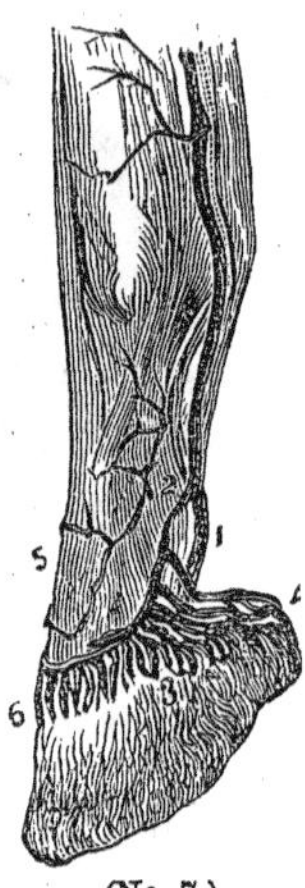

(No. 7.)

View of Vessels of th Foot, injected.

1. Plantar vein.
2. Plantar artery.
3. Branches to th coronary substanc and laminæ.
4. Posterior divi sion of plantar ar tery.
5. Perpendicula branch.
6. Anastomosi with opposite plan tar artery.

The healthy foot is the best model for guidance, and the object should be in preparing the foot for the shoe, to simply bring it back to its natural form, and bearing. If the toe is too long, or the heels too high, or there is an unusual accumulation of old horn on the sole, remove so much as will restore the foot to its natural proportions and bearing.

If the shoes have been on a month, cut away the horn grown more or less, according to the length of time the shoes have been on and the quantity of horn grown. If the foot is in a healthy condition, it is seldom necessary to interfere with the sole and frog. The sole and frog throw off horn by a natural process of expoliation; but sometimes the shoe extends so close and so far over the sole as to prevent this old horn from either wearing or scaling off. When this is the case, it should be dressed out, particularly at the heels, at the angles formed between the bars and crust. The buttress is usually so large and square edged as to make it unsuitable for doing this. Even with the greatest care, it is difficult, with such an instrument, to prevent cutting away too much at some points, while there cannot be enough cut away at others. An English shave, with the end turned back, like that of an instrument with which to mark boards, is just the thing for this purpose. While the object, in the first place, should be to reduce the hoof to its natural size, care should be used not to cut away too much of the wall; for, bear in mind, cutting away too much must bring the shoe against the sole, and forces driving the nails too deep into the wall of the hoof, if not into the vascular part, inside, which would not only cause lameness, but be liable to induce the secretion of matter, and very serious consequences would follow. (See Causes of Lameness.) And besides, forcing so many nails into this thin horn weakens it so much that by a few repetitions of such shoeing it becomes difficult to nail on shoes with any certainty of being held to the foot very long, and, of course, the more re-nailing the more the mischief is increased.

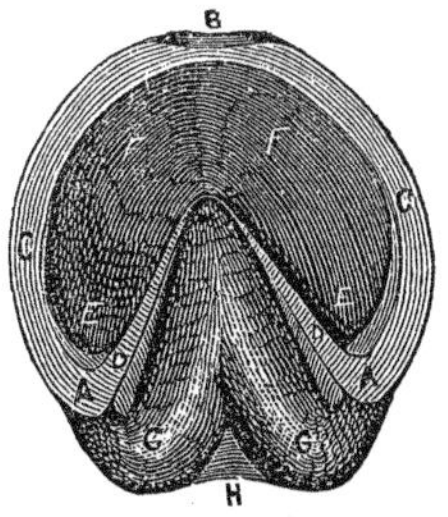

(No. 8.)

A Sound Fore-foot, prepared for the Shoe.

a The heel of the crust. *b* The toe cut out to receive the clip. *c c* The quarters of the crust. *d d* The bars as they should be left, with the full frog between them. *e e* The angles between the heel and bars, where corns appear. *f f* The concave surface of the toe. *g g* The bulbous heels. *h* The cleft.

The bearing surface should be leveled down carefully and left a little higher than the sole, so that there can be no bearing of the sole upon the shoe. If the foot is flat and will not bear this, then the shoe must be lowered inside of the part coming under the wall, so that the sole will not touch it. No definite rule can be given by which to explain just how much to cut away, or the limit. If the heels are strong and upright, they should be cut down so that the bearing will be level and the hoof appear natural. (See cut 8.)

The next aim is to form and fit the shoe so as to approximate it to the size and bearing of the foot and work of the horse. If the hoof is thin shelled and the horse is not worked much, the shoe should be light; but if the work is hard, more weight will be necessary. No general rule will apply here. The shoer is to understand that if the foot is properly prepared as directed, the shoe must be made big enough to just come out even with the edge of the hoof from the toe to the turn of the heels, becoming a little wider at the extremity of the heels, for as the foot enlarges by growth, the shoe is brought forward under the heels until it loses its original proportion and becomes too short and narrow, to allow for which the shoe should be as much wider and longer than the foot at the heels (about a quarter of an inch) as it is supposed the foot will grow in the time it is intended to keep the shoes on before being re-set. The bearing surface of the shoe should be perfectly level, and only so much of the shoe as comes under the wall of the hoof should touch the foot. Either the foot must be prepared so that the shoe cannot come down to the sole, or that part of the shoe coming inside the wall of the hoof must be so hammered down that the sole cannot possibly touch the shoe. (See cuts 8 and 9.)

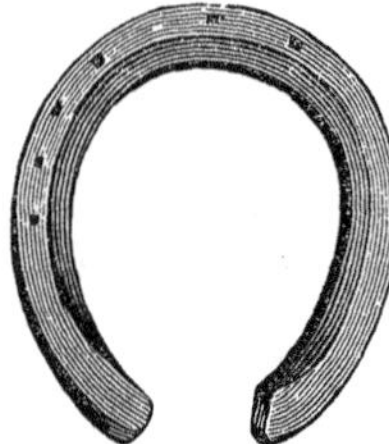

(No. 9.) Shoe, inner surface beveled to prevent contact with Sole of Foot.

This requires being exact, no guessing or coming "pretty near" the thing and nailing on. The shoe should be so fitted that when laid on a level surface every part of the bearing surface would touch, and it should fit equally well to the foot.

If the shoe as usually fitted is examined, the bearing surface

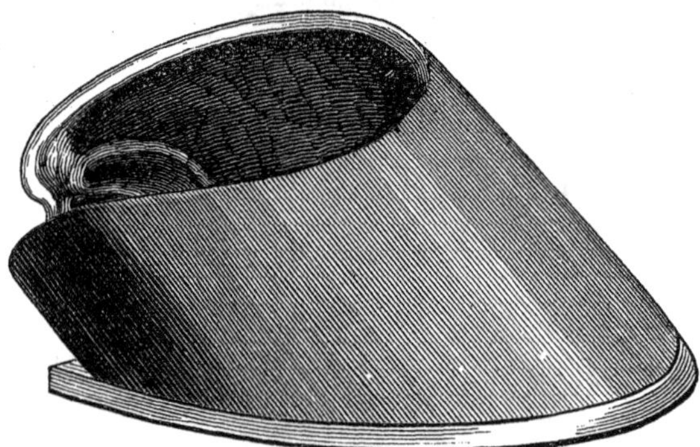

(No. 10.) Shoe Properly Fitted.

at the heels will be found concave or the inner edge of each heel much the lowest; not only this, but often the heels are carried back too far, or the shoe is so wide that the heels rest on the seating inside of where fitted to support the heels.

It is evident that if the bearing surface at the heels is concave, there is a natural tendency as weight is thrown upon the foot to have the heels crowded together.

With the foot properly prepared and the shoe properly fitted to it, the next important consideration is nailing it to the hoof. As the hoof is continually growing and becoming proportionately larger than the shoe, this must be done if possible so as not to bring lateral restraint upon the quarters, and this implies attention to the location of the nail holes. If the smith were to examine the thickness of the hoof of an ordinary

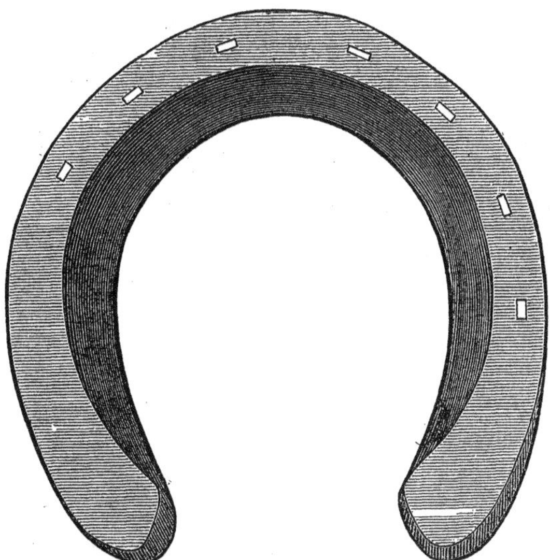

(No. 11.) Bearing Surface Level.

well-bred horse, he would perhaps be surprised at its thinness, and he would see the importance, in the first place, of making the holes near the edge well forward in the toe, and of not putting the shoe so far under the shell as to compel his driving the nails too deeply into it, or of having the nails so large as to split and shatter the hoof. If the nail holes are made well into the shoe, and the shoe should be a little narrow or short, and be set well under the hoof, the nails must be driven very near, or into the quick, which must result in serious lameness or injury. Two points, therefore, must be kept in view by the smith in punching the nail holes. First, making them so far forward in the toe as to prevent needless restraint upon the quarters. Second, so near the edge of the shoe as not to endanger driving the nails too deep in the crust. The nails should not be large, nor a greater number driven than is barely necessary to retain the shoe.

It must be remembered that, at best, the hoof is greatly shattered by the nails; that the horn is thickest at the toe,

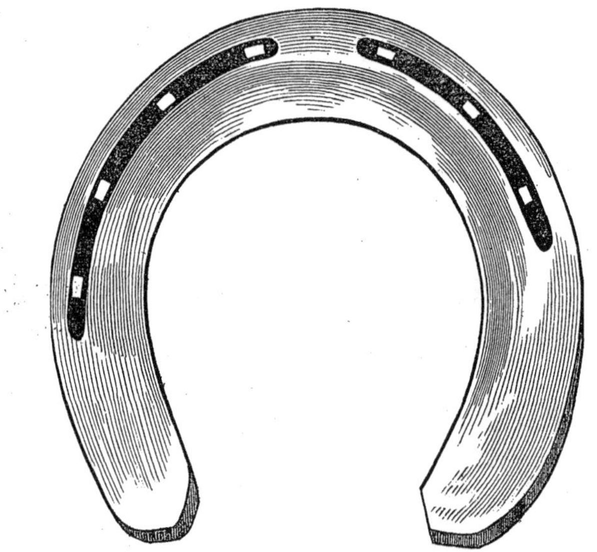

(No. 12.) Ground Surface—Position of Nails.

and the nailing well back to the quarters not only exposes to greater danger of pricking, but causes an injurious pressure upon the heels. If the horse is not used much, and the heels are rather square and upright, the quarters must be kept free. Have the nail holes made well forward on both sides, three on the inner and four on the outer side, or nail well back on the outside quarter, but well forward in the toe inside. As the foot now grows, the shoe will be carried to that side and forward, leaving the inside quarter free, thereby making both quarters as independent of the restraint of the shoe as it is possible to do. Any increase in the number of nails to retain the shoe more firmly must not imply freedom to drive them back in the quarters. Let the holes be punched closer together in the toe. Care should be used not to file too deeply nnder the clinches, as is common; and in finishing off, the file should not be touched above the clinches, and below only enough to round the toe a little. There is a *penchant* in most smiths to improve the shape of the foot by rasping and filing the whole surface to the hair. The outside of the hoof is much more dense and hard than the inside, the small spaces between the fibres of the horn are filled with a soft substance—the better to prevent a too rapid evaporation of moisture. If the whole surface of the hoof is rasped, the best part is not only likely to be cut away, but too rapid evaporation takes place, and the hoof is not only thereby weakened, but becomes dry, hard and contracted. If the horse is not used much, and stands on dry plank, this condition must be produced.

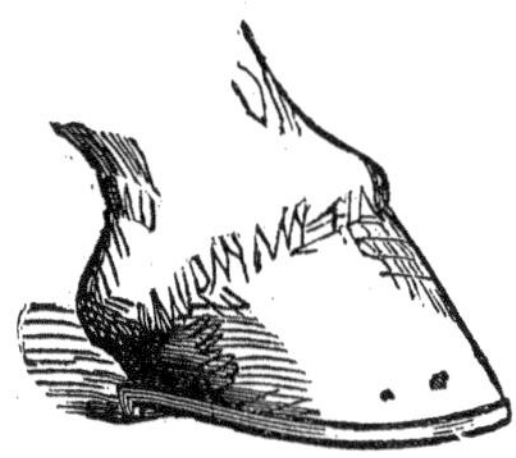

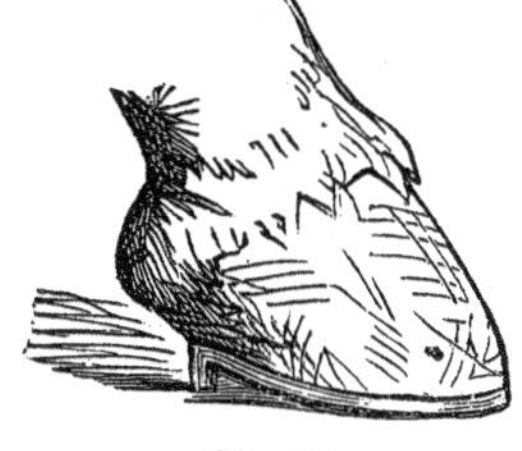

(No. 13.) (No. 14.)

Foot properly shod, and a foot that has been rasped down too much, in order to fit the shoe, which is too small for it.

There is a very grave fault in the fitting and nailing of shoes, namely: if they happen to be too short, of setting them well back from the toe, which not only necessitates driving the nails so deep into the hoof as to prick and lame the animal, but also destroys the proportion of the foot by cutting down the toe too much. (See cuts 13 and 14.) Smiths seem to think it necessary to cut the hoof down to the shoe, no matter how far under the shell it may be. This is wrong, as the shoe is now pressing upon and nailed to the inside or soft part of the shell, which of itself leads to soreness and derangement. (See cuts 9 and 10.) In the first place the hoof should not be cut away too much in preparing for the shoe, but should leave plenty of strong, hard horn, through which to nail. In the second place, the shoe should come out even with the hoof; and third, the nails should be driven deep enough to hold firmly. Some shoers have a

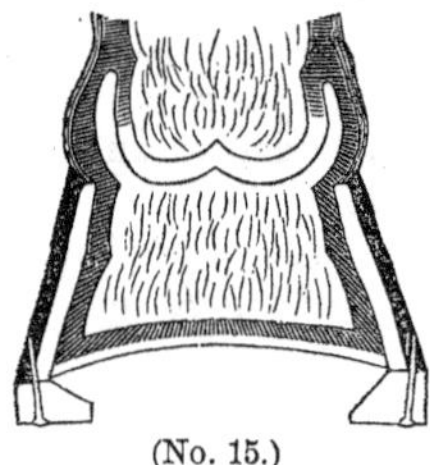

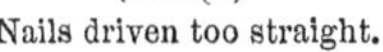

(No. 15.)
Nails driven too straight.

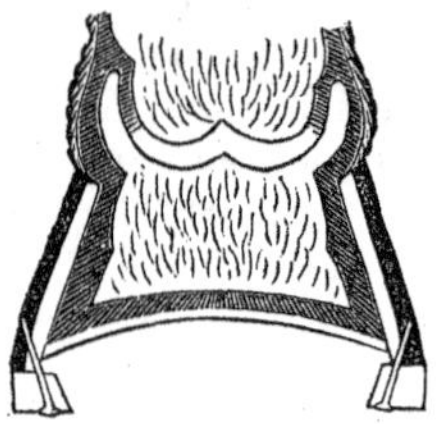

(No, 16.)
How to nail the Shoe.

faculty of going from one extreme to the other by driving the nails so near the outer edge of the crust that there is almost certainty of breaking through. (See cuts 15 and 16.) Illustrative of this see cut 15; the hold of the nail is not deep enough; whereas in 16 the nail is started deep and comes out low, getting a good, strong hold, and not endangering driving into the quick. There should be no effort to cut down the hoof in any way that would weaken it, or destroy its natural appearance and bearing.

Contraction of the Feet.

If we examine the foot in its natural, healthy state, it will be found almost round, and very elastic at the heel. The frog, broad, plump, and of a soft, yielding character. The commissures open and well defined, and the sole concave. The outside of the crust, from the heel to the toe, increased from a slight bevel to an angle of about forty-five degrees. In a state of contraction the heels are narrow and high, the commissures closed and the frog small, and from bad shoeing a marked change in size and form. Corns, or bruising of the sole at the heels, or any difficulty causing lameness, is induced by inflammation. Now, any cause by which the sensible sole or muscular structure uniting the coffin-bone to the wall of the hoof is bruised and inflamed, leads to either decomposition and the formation of matter, thickening of cartilage, or growth of unnatural bony matter.

The most common cause of inflammation, producing change of structure and lameness, is contraction. It is evident that the more horn is grown the wider and longer the foot becomes, and the more cut away the narrower and shorter it is made. If a shoe be fitted accurately to a foot after being trimmed and prepared carefully, it would be found in a few weeks to be much too short and narrow or too small for the same foot.

The foot is continually growing and losing its original proportions with the shoe, which in four or five weeks becomes at least a quarter of an inch wider and longer than it was when dressed. Now there must be not only special provision made in nailing for this increased enlargement, but the greatest care should be used not to permit any lateral, mechanical pressure upon the quarters that would restrict their freedom.

It must be observed that shoeing first raises the frog from contact with the ground, which, of itself, removes an important auxiliary to health in the foot; second, that nailing the shoe to the sides of the hoof brings direct restraint upon the quarters with increased force, and to the degree that this nailing is extended to the heels and the foot increases in size by growth, is the foot contracted by the restraint thus unavoidably produced.

There also is another cause of derangement requiring special notice, namely: the bearing surface at the heels is usually inclined inward, or the inside edge is much lower than the outer edge, often quite or more than a sixteenth of an inch, which alone is sufficient to cause serious contraction. In addition to which the increased absorption of moisture, induced both by inflammation and by keeping the feet dry, tends directly to this end, since the dryer and harder horn becomes, the more lessened in size. Of course, if direct pressure is brought upon the foot by which the vascular structure beneath the shell is bruised and inflamed, lameness and ultimate change of structure must ensue, which, if permitted, may cause serious or even incurable lameness.

There is one peculiarity about contraction that seems to puzzle even good practitioners, which is the increased growth of the heels. The heels grow down rapidly, and the shell becomes very thick, while the frog becomes small and hard. If cut No. 16 is examined the sole will be seen to be arched. Now it is evident if the quarters are pressed together this bending of the sole upward is increased, bringing increased pressure upon the suspensory ligaments and coffin-joint, and force the coffin-joint upwards and forward against the hoof at its upper edge.

Now if you look at cut No. 5, you will discover an artery passing down on each side of the leg. which divides above the hoof into two branches, one forward around the edge of the hoof, and another back to the heel, which again throw off innumerable branches. The office of these arteries is to supply material for the growth of horn. Now the pressure induced upon the coffin-bone by the pressing of the sole against it as before explained, forces the coffin-bone against the upper edge of the hoof, and thus presses directly upon this artery, thereby obstructing the flow of blood to this part, and forcing it back into those supplying horn at the heels. Hence the forward part of the hoof grows slowly and becomes thin, while the heels grow down rapidly, becoming high and thick.

The first and important object in curing disease is, to remove the cause. We must do more than this in the cure of contraction by removing the surplus horn accumulated and applying mechanical pressure in such a way as to gradually spread the foot back to its natural form and condition as it will bear.

To do this we must first thoroughly soften the feet by poulticing. Next cut down the heels to within an eighth of an inch or a little more of the line yielding horn of the sole, trimming out the sole thoroughly. Cut down carefully between the bars and frog. If not careful you will cut through and bring blood at the extreme of the heel, while you have not cut deep enough farther forward. Follow the curve of the sole, aiming to cut out an average depth until the heels will yield easily to a little pressure.

The next object is to gradually force the heels outward. There are three ways of doing this:

First, form the shoe of an equal thickness all the way round, with nail holes punched well back in the heels, and fit accurately to the foot, so that it will come out even with the edge of the hoof. Now drive the nails carefully, so that they will be deep enough into the horn to hold firmly without endangering pricking, leaving the points stick down straight. After all are driven down, pull them out again. Heat the shoe and spread it about one-eighth of an inch, more or less according to what the foot will bear, and put on again. Now, drive the nails again, each a little at a time until driven home, and clinch firmly. It is seen that the shoe must now exert an outward pressure upon the heels equal to the increased breadth of the shoe. Keep the foot reasonably soft. In a few days or a week the clinches can be carefully drawn, the nails pulled out, the shoe made wider and nailed as before, which can be repeated so long as the nails will hold well.

A simpler method is that of the convex shoe, (cut 17.) The foot is prepared as before, with the difference of not cutting away the bearing surface so much at the heels. The shoe, instead of having the bearing surface level, should be made convex, the outer edge from an eighth to three-sixteenths of an inch lower than the inner edge, running out at the toe. This surface should be filed down carefully, and so fitted to the foot that the heels will rest on these inclined surfaces, the shoe being a little wider than the heels, and nail on. Now there is a continued slipping outward of the heels when weight is thrown upon the foot. Remember one point here. Do not commit the error of cutting down the heels very close. You must have horn enough to keep the shoe from possibly coming in contact with the sole. If it does, the inner edge pressing upon the sole forms a shoulder which will not only prevent expansion, but bring pressure upon the yielding sole, bruising the sensitive sole above, and acute lameness will result.

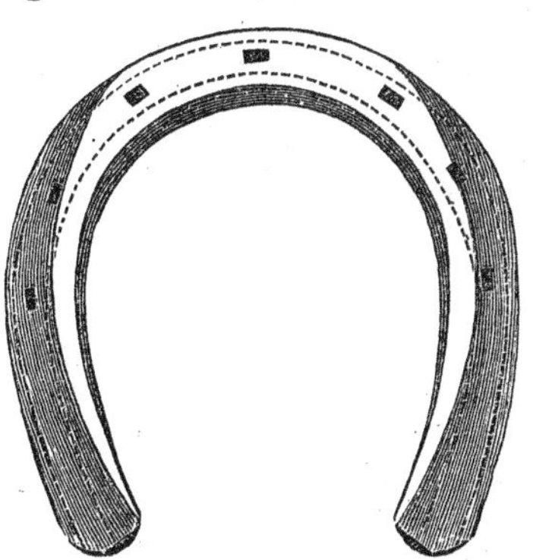

(No. 17.) Convex Shoe for the cure of Contraction.

The third, and by far the best, is that of Tyrrel's patent shoe, (cut 18.) By this shoe, if properly fitted and applied, the foot can be expanded as little or as much as may be desired. It will also enable expanding one or both heels as may be desired, and is unquestionably the best form of shoe ever invented for the cure of contraction. The only difference there is in this shoe from the common form is: first, the inside edges of the heels are turned up into little clips; second, the shoe is so cut out at each side of the toe as to enable bending the quarters outward, by putting the tongs or a screw between the heels and pressing them outward. The clips at the heels extending up inside of the bars at the extreme of the heels press the heels outward just so much as the shoe is spread, which can be done every few days at will until the foot is expanded as much as may be desired. This is the great consideration in the cure of contractions so far as mechanical pressure is concerned, and of all the shoes I have seen for the purpose, this is the best, and in my judgment is unrivaled. With its use contraction can be cured in a short time. This shoe has been thoroughly tested, and is shown to be the best for the cure of contracted feet ever brought into use. Gentlemen desiring shoes of this form, with full instructions in relation to their application and permission of use, must address the owners, TYRREL & FERREN, Batavia, New York.

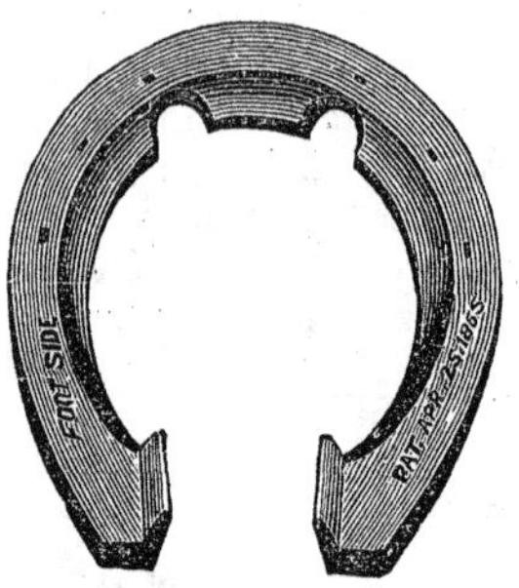

(No. 18.) Tyrrel's Patent Shoe for the cure of Contraction.

This shoe is also the very best for the cure of splitting of the hoof, as it enables pressure upon the quarters outward, and thus keeps the parts pressed together.

Corns

Appear in the angle of the hoof near the heel. They are generally caused by the shoe being worn too long, causing the shell of the hoof to grow over the shoe, which throws the weight upon the sole, or the angles between the bar and crust are not properly dressed out. If the descending heel of the coffin bone meets with too much resistance by want of elasticity in the sole at this place, the sensitive sole is liable to be so bruised and injured as to produce corns, which are simply a contused wound of the sensitive sole. If of an ordinary character, upon cutting away the horn, there will be found a red spot; if very bad, the color will be a dark purple and deeper seated.

If in this condition it is neglected, matter may be formed, or the inflammation may cause the lateral cartilages which are attached to the heels of the coffin bone to become ossified, or even the accumulation of large, bony deposits, which would destroy the mobility of the foot and cause considerable deformity.

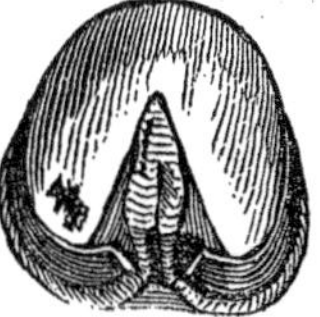

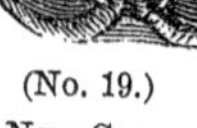

(No. 19.)
New Corn.

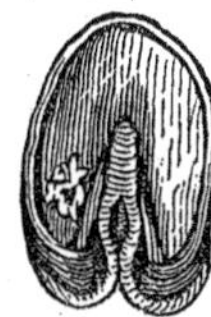

(No. 20.)
Situation and appearance of an old corn.

All pressure must be removed from the part. First, dress down the part bruised until quite thin. Put a little sulphur on, and burn in pretty well with a hot iron, or put on buttyr of antimony, which will stimulate a healthy growth of horn.

If there is much inflammation, poultice; and if there is a cavity or the sensible sole is exposed, put on a little pitch and tallow, over which spread a little tow. Put on the shoe so fitted there will be no pressure on the part. To do this a bar shoe will often be necessary. (See cut No. 22.) The shoe should be re-set frequently until cured.

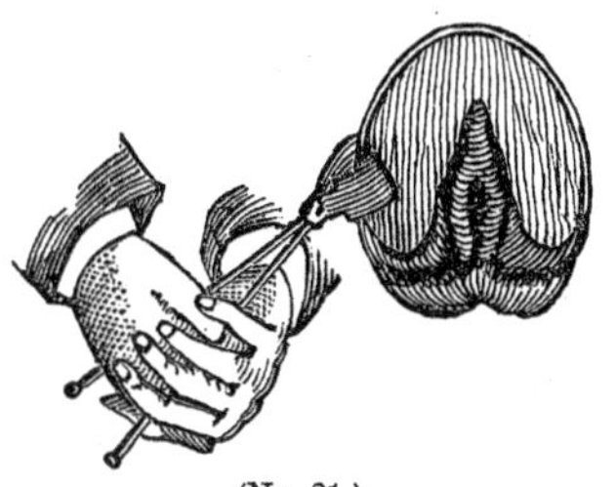

(No. 21.)
Testing for Corns.

Quarter Crack.

When the hoof is dry and hard it is easily split. A piece of glue when very dry splits and breaks very easily if pounded upon, but if softened by moisture would only bend and be bruised. The hoof partakes of the character of glue. If very dry the fibres become dense and hard. If while the feet are in this condition the horse is driven fast on hard roads, the hoof is liable to burst. If the hoof is thin and contracted, there is great danger of the inside quarters splitting.

Cut down the hoof back of the crack, so that there is no pressure of that part of the bearing surface upon the shoe, put on a bar shoe, cut across the split deeply at the edge of the hair with a firing iron. Next cut down the edges of the hoof so far as split extends, to the quick. Then soften and grow down the hoof rapidly by applying any good, stimulating ointment. A mixture of equal portions of tar, lard and turpentine, is excellent for this purpose. The fitting of the shoe should be carefully attended to, the hoof grown down as rapidly as it is safe to do, and the part kept clean by covering it with a little tar, or a mixture of resin and tallow. There will not be a cure until a new hoof is grown down, which will take about six or eight months.

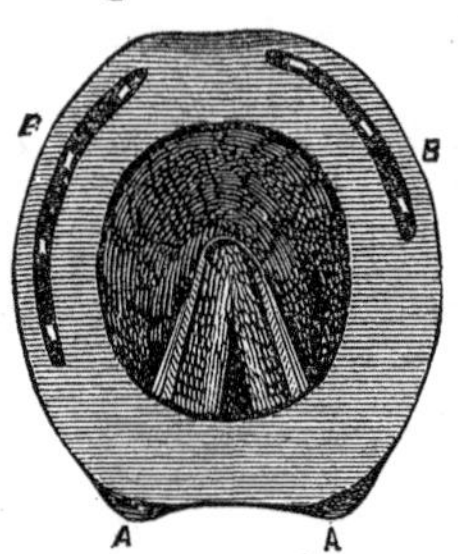

(No. 22.)
Bar Shoe for Corns.

Interfering.

Some horses travel so close that the least neglect of having the shoe well under the quarter, and the part nicely dressed down, would cause a bruising and cutting of the opposite ankle. If you do not know what part of the hoof strikes the ankle, wind the ankle with a piece of bandage and daub it with some coloring matter; then trot the horse until some of this coloring is found on the hoof, which indicates the part that strikes. The shoe should be so formed and fitted as to come well under this portion of the hoof. To do this well, that side of the shoe should be made rather straight, with the web narrow, and the nail-holes well forward in the toe; at all events there must be no nails driven into that part of the hoof that strikes, as the clinches will be likely to cut. If the toe-*cork* is set well round, on the inside of the toe, and the foot is so pared, or the shoe is so formed that the bearing of the inside of the foot is raised somewhat, there will be a tending in the ankle to be thrown out when borne upon. But the great object is to have the shoe fitted and filed smoothly, and set well under the part hitting, so that after the

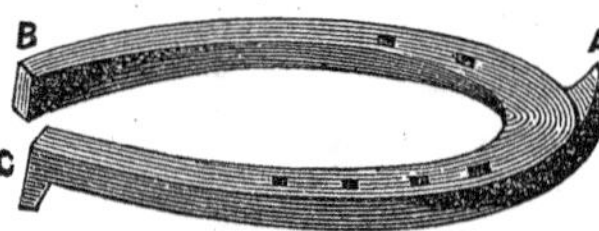

(No. 23.)
Interfering Shoe.

hoof is rasped off all it is prudent to do, and rounded down carefully, the shoe sets far enough under not to endanger its cutting, yet supports the hoof, and gives a natural bearing to the foot. The chief danger will be that some portion of this part of the shoe, will be made to extend beyond the hoof, and the shoe be fitted and put on so roughly that it can scarcely be said to be fitted any smoother or better than is usually done, without regard to such a purpose. It is always best to keep the bearing natural by trimming the foot level, and making the shoe of an even thickness, but set it under and file smoothly. If this will not do, raise the inside a little. Driving young horses to sulky will often cause interfering; getting a horse in good condition will often overcome the difficulty. If the ankles are cut or sore, they should be protected with pads until well. If the owner values the animal highly, he should give such shoeing his personal attention.

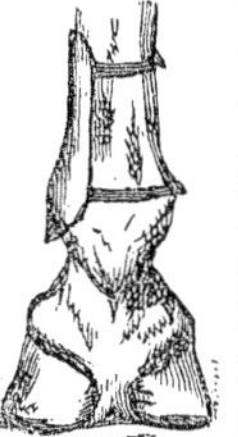

(No. 24.)
Interfering Pad.

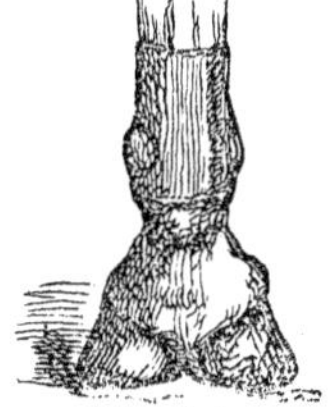

(No. 25.)
A Leather Boot to protect the Ankle.

Pricking.

If the smith should happen to drive a nail so deep into the crust as to strike the sensitive part, he should by no means drive a nail into that hole again, so that if matter is formed by the injury there will be an outlet for it. If the horse becomes lame after being shod, examine the foot carefully. If pricked by driving any of the nails too near the quick, there will be heat and tenderness in the hoof easily discovered. Have the shoe taken off, and cut down to where the nail strikes the quick, enough to make room for any matter that may have formed to escape; then poultice with flax seed meal until the inflammation is reduced, when a little tar, resin, or tallow, or something of this kind, should be put on, and the opening filled up with a little tow to prevent gravel or dirt from getting in, and the shoe put on again.

Weak Heels.

Cutting down too close and fitting the shoes roughly, so that the horse wears and breaks down the heels, will cause them to be low and sensitive. Such feet should be simply leveled down with the rasp carefully, and the shoe fitted to touch every part of the bearing surface at the heels.

Shoes.

It should be borne in mind that that form of shoe which accords with the foot in making the bearing natural, preserves its elasticity and protects it from injury, is best. If we examine the foot it will be found concave. This is the best form to enable a fulcrum that will prevent slipping. If we would imitate and carry out in the form of the shoe, that of the foot, it should be also concave, or thick at the outer edge and beveled upward to the inner edge on the ground surface. Such a shoe will not ball, prevents slipping, is lighter, and would certainly enable more speed on a track if at all wet. *Amateurs who have an opportunity should see my models of shoes of different patterns.*

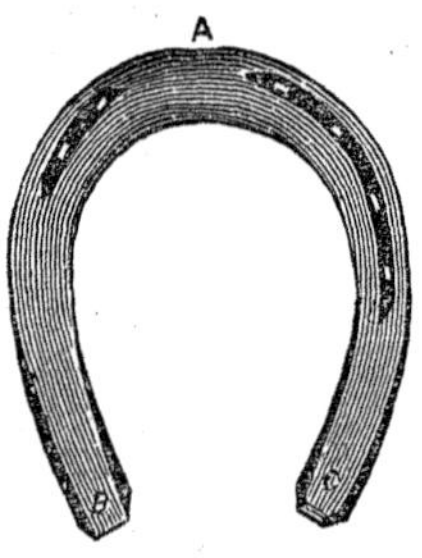

(No. 26.)

Shoes for summer wear should be level, of an equal thickness from toe to heel. If the roads are soft, this is certainly advisable, to give the frog pressure. If shoes are made with corks, the inside ones should be rounded, so as not to cut the feet. The outside ones will prevent slipping. My "Maine Snow Shoe" is undoubtedly the best for winter use; will not ball, and prevents the feet most effectually from being bruised or injured.

The bearing surface of all shoes should be level, and come exactly under the wall of the hoof all the way round. The nails should be as small, and as few, and as far forward in the toe as will retain the shoe safely, the object being to protect the foot and keep it healthy. When from any cause there is an undue absorption of moisture, making the frog and hoof dry and hard, either from inactivity by standing on a dry floor, or driving on dry hard roads, or both, it must be supplied by artificial means. Stuff or fill the feet with flax-seed meal, to which has been added a little wood ashes mixed with water. It will stick. Or wet cloths may be tied around the hoof.

If there is soreness of the feet, put them in water as hot as can be borne, for an hour each day, for one or two weeks, or blister mildly around the coronet, repeated two or three times.

If there is a dry, hard condition of the feet, apply moisture around the coronet by tieing wet cloths around the hoof, or poulticing, stopping the feet with flaxseed meal, as before explained; after which, apply some of the preparation for softening the feet and stimulating the growth of horn.

The usual palliative means of rubber cushions and such means, put between the hoof, to cure soreness and lameness, are of no account, since they do not reach the cause of difficulty. The nailing of the shoe must necessarily be so tight as to press out all the elasticity there is, and, in addition, the heels cut through such means so quickly that they will not prove of any real value.

Shoes should be re-set once in from four to six weeks. For light, occasional use, not more than seven nails should be driven—four on the outside and three on the inside—well forward. The shoe should come well out under the toe, so that there is no necessity for more than touching the edge a little to reach the shoe, and by all means do not allow that reckless rasping of the outside of the hoof so general with shoers. If the shoe is short it should not be a reason that the hoof must be cut down to it. Even rasping under the clinches should not be permitted. A thin shell can be easily ruined in this way; besides, this rasping of the whole surface of the hoof not only removes the strongest and hardest part, but permits too rapid an evaporation, which causes the horn to become hard and brittle. It is much better, easier and cheaper to *keep* the feet healthy than to *cure* them. It is wise in shoers to be patient and do the work well, and owners should remember that extra care and skill deserves extra compensation. It is hoped that the few explanations given will aid in a better understanding of this duty.

If the horse shows sudden lameness in the foot, especially after being shod, examine it carefully; strike the hoof lightly with a small hammer; put the hand first on one foot and then on the other, that you may discover any increased heat. If a nail has been driven too deep, remove the shoe. If much inflammation, poultice—usually necessary for twenty-four hours or more—when cover the part with tow and a preparation of tar and resin, or pitch and common grease. If a nail has been driven into the foot, get the horse to the stable as quick as you can, take off the shoe, poultice the foot, and give a sharp dose of physic, and let the animal stand quietly. The object is to keep down inflammation. No hot oils or anything stimulating is to be applied.

I would by all means keep the wound wet with *callendula*, which should be reduced one-half by adding soft water. Second best treatment, *digestive ointment.* Next, any of the digestive remedies. There is liable to be tenderness if the sole should strike the ground afterwards, as there may be inflammation of the periosteum, to relieve which, put on a high-heeled shoe and blister around the coronet. The sole is sometimes bruised by the shoe pressing upon it, causing much inflammation and lameness. Take off the shoe, poultice for twenty-four hours or more; fit the shoe so as to remove all pressure from the sole; if sore yet, continue the poultice; if matter is formed, treat as you would any such ulcer, with a healing astringent. Several good preparations are given in another part of this work.

DISEASES AND THEIR TREATMENT.

THE treatment and remedies given in the following pages can be used with confidence. While the treatment given is the very best, there are many special remedies, of the greatest value, never before published, worth from ten to fifty dollars each to any horseman. The author has spent thousands of dollars and much valuable time (devoting one year to special study and practice with one of the best veterinary surgeons in the United States) in acquiring the knowledge imparted here, besides including all the favorite remedies, prized for their great curative powers, gathered by him, at a large cost, during his long experience before the public in his profession.

Colic—Spasmodic and Flatulent.

Colic is one of the most common as well as most dangerous diseases to which the horse is subject. There are two forms of this disease, namely, Spasmodic and Flatulent Colic.

The first is wholly of a spasmodic nature, and if not relieved, will, in severe cases, run into inflammation of the bowels, causing speedy death.

The second, while exhibiting the same general symptoms, shows marked enlargement of the belly, from generation of gas, which, if not checked and neutralized, results fatally by rupturing the diaphram, causing suffocation and death.

I will first give the simplest and safest treatment for each; after which I will include a remedy which is almost a specific for both, and cannot be too highly prized.

The common causes of colic are, application of cold water to the body, drinking cold water when in a heated condition, costiveness, unwholesome food, &c.

First—*Spasmodic Colic.* Premonitory symptoms are sudden. The animal paws violently, showing evidences of great distress, shifting his position almost constantly, and manifest-

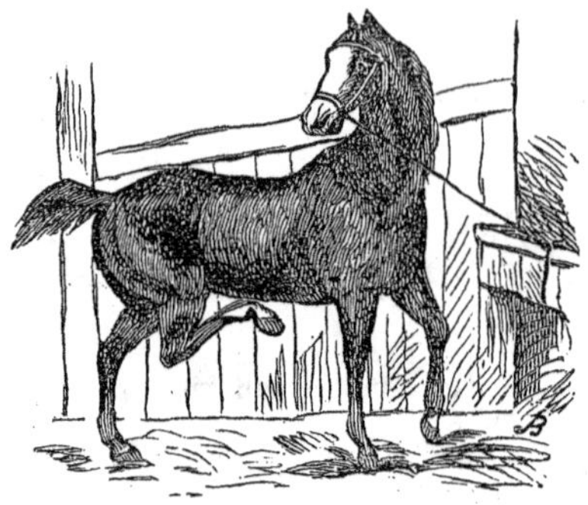

First Stage of Spasmodic Colic.

ing a desire to lie down. In a few minutes these symptoms disappear, and the horse is easy. But the same uneasiness soon returns, increasing in severity until the animal cannot be kept upon his feet; the pulse is full, scarcely altered from its normal condition; a cold sweat breaks out over the body; temperature of legs and ears natural. As the disease advances the symptoms become more severe, the animal at times throwing himself down with force, regardless of consequences, looks anxiously at the sides, sometimes snapping with the teeth at the sides, looking anxiously at the belly, and striking upward with the hind feet, showing almost the same symptoms as in inflammation of the bowels. There are, however, strongly marked characteristics peculiar to each. The better to point them out, I will tabulate them, by which the difference and peculiarities of each can be easily determined.

COLIC.	INFLAMMATION OF BOWELS.
Sudden in its attacks.	Gradual in its approach, with previous indications of fever.
Pulse, in the early stage of the disease, not much quickened or altered in its character.	*Pulse* much quickened, small, and often scarcely to be felt.
Legs and ears of a natural temperature.	Legs and ears cold.
Rubbing the belly gives relief.	Belly very tender and painful to the touch.
Relief obtained from motion.	Motion increases pain.
Intervals of rest.	Constant pain.
Strength scarcely affected.	Rapid and great weakness.

This disease being wholly of a spasmodic nature, it must be counteracted by antispasmodic treatment; bleeding being the most powerful method of relaxing the system, taking from six to twelve quarts of blood from the neck vein, more or less, according to the size of the horse and severity of the case. Always in bleeding make the orifice large and extract the blood as quickly as possible.

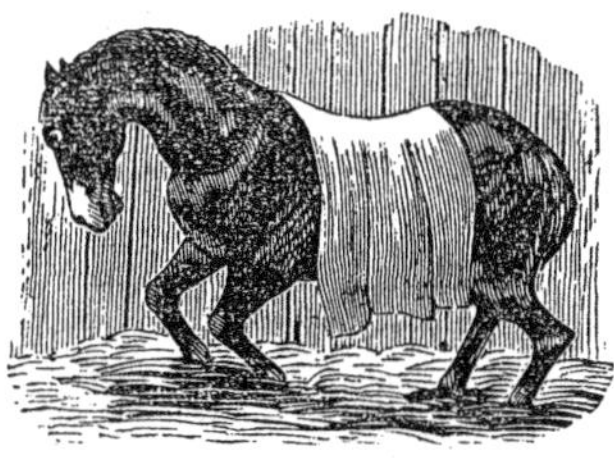
Second Stage of Spasmodic Colic.

If not bled, give from two to three ounces of laudanum and a pint of raw linseed oil. If not better in an hour, give two ounces of laudanum and the same quantity of oil.

The peppermint and ether, as recommended for flatulent colic, will sometimes work admirably in this, and may be tried at first, if at hand.

Aconite, belledonna, colocynth and nux vomica, in doses of from five to ten drops, in a little water or sugar, given upon the tongue, repeated every fifteen or twenty minutes, will often cure colic promptly. This is homeopathic treatment, and is very good.

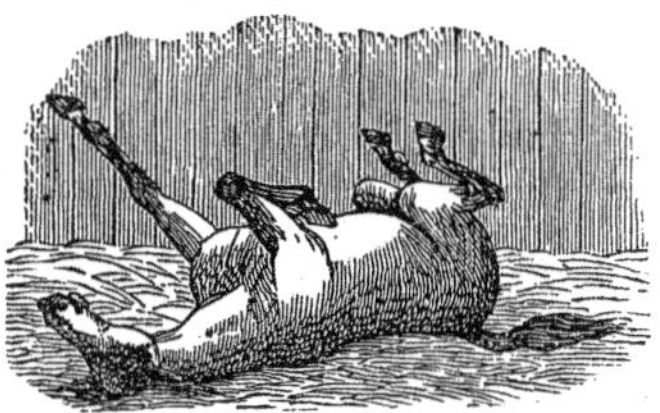
Third Stage of Spasmodic Colic.

Flatulent Colic, (Tympanites.)

Symptoms same as spasmodic colic, with the difference of there being so great an accumulation of gas in the stomach and intestines that the belly is swelled. This disease will often prove fatal in from one to three hours. It is generally very sudden in its attack, often occurring while the animal is at work, particularly during warm weather or changeable weather from cold to heat; but is generally caused by indigestion, producing gases in the stomach or bowels. The horse is violently swollen along the belly, flanks and side generally. There are sometimes belchings of gas through the

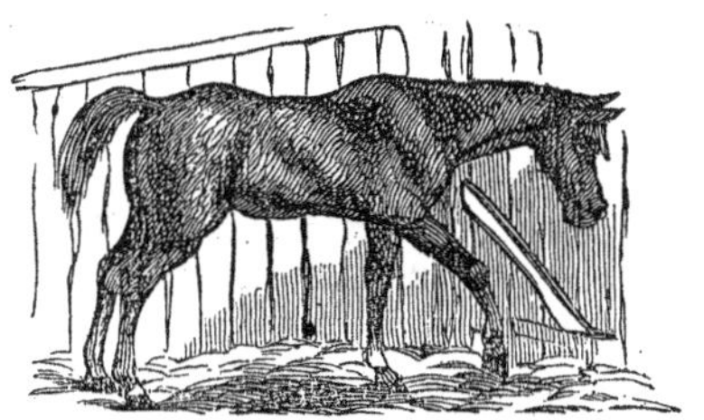
First Stage of Flatulent Colic.

esophagus or gullet. Pulse is rarely disturbed until the disease advances, when it will become quickened, running to its height rapidly, and receding as quickly if fatal. If to terminate fatally, it will become weaker and slower until it is almost imperceptible.

In this case, bleeding must not be attempted, neither must any fluids be forced into the rectum. The animal loses strength rapidly, and to bleed prostrates too much and checks perspiration, without lessening accumulation of gas, and death must almost surely follow.

Treatment.—Blanket warmly, in order to keep up perspiration as much as possible, and give the following immediately: Two ounces sulphuric ether, two ounces peppermint, one pint of water; to be taken at one dose. If not relieved, repeat in thirty or forty minutes. Keep the animal as quiet as possible, and give a good bed to lie on.

Note.—The ether disturbs the breathing, making the horse apparently distressed—breathes laboriously—but will pass off in a few hours.

If much bloated, do not let the horse lie down, as the shock might cause the diaphram to be ruptured, when of course all hope of saving the animal would result only in disappointment.

The above treatment is the best and most reliable perhaps ever used for this dangerous disease. I have never known it to fail when given in a reasonable time.

It is seldom necessary to repeat the dose more than once to cure.

ANOTHER GOOD REMEDY FOR COLIC.

The following remedy, if at hand, will be found invaluable for the cure of *spasmodic* or *flatulent colic.* It will afford almost immediate relief if given soon after commencement of attack, and is almost a specific for this dangerous disease:

Sulphuric ether, 1 pint; aromatic spirits ammonia, 1 pint; sweet spirits nitre, 2 pints; opium, ¼ lb.; asafœtida, (pure,) ½ lb.; camphor, ½ lb. Put it in a large bottle, let it stand fourteen days, with frequent shaking, and it will be fit to use. Dose: One ounce, more or less, according to the severity of the case, once in from thirty minutes to an hour. Should be given in a little water, which may be sweetened.

Owners of valuable horses should keep a supply of this medicine on hand ready for use.

Inflammation of the Lungs.

Any cause by which the circulation is obstructed and deranged may excite inflammation of the lungs. The most common are, exposing the animal while warm to a cold wind, or becoming chilled from driving fast against a cold wind, washing with cold water immediately after exercise, changes from heat to cold, or from cold to heat, removing from a warm to a cold or from a cold to a warm stable, or cold applied to the surface of a heated animal, by which the blood is driven from the skin and extremities to the internal organs, may cause inflammation of the lungs (pneumonia), pleurisy, congestion of the lungs, inflammation of the bowels (enterilis), founder (laminitis), or other difficulties of a similar nature.

When the lungs are involved, the severity or mildness of the attack and the part inflamed indicates the extreme and character of the disease. Thus: When the pleuro, a membrane that surrounds the lungs and extends between them and the walls of the chest, is inflamed, the disease is called pleurisy. When the inflammation is located in the lungs, it is called *pneumonia*, or inflammation of the lungs. When the action of the capillaries is greatly lessened from their being weakened, or the blood being so forced through them that they are obstructed and clogged, the difficulty is called *congestion* of the lungs.

There cannot be inflammation of a part without there being more or less inflammation of the other parts surrounding, and there cannot be inflammation without congestion, as there is always obstruction of the circulation where there is inflammation.

As pleurisy, inflammation of the lungs and congestion of the lungs are only different types of the same disease, excited by the same general causes, and the treatment for each is almost the same, I will include their treatment under the same general head. The better, however, to guide the reader, I will give the symptoms of each.

PLEURISY

may be sudden or gradual in its attack, the horse showing indisposition sometimes for days previous. The horse will be dull and heavy in action for a day or two, unwilling to lie down, pulse not much disturbed, or there is a chill, which lasts from one to three hours, when fever sets in; breathing at flanks a little accelerated, countenance is anxious, the head is sometimes turned towards the side, does not lie down. As the disease advances the symptoms become more marked. The ears and legs become cold; the pulse, from being a little accelerated, grows quicker, hard and full; the head is hung forward, stands up persistently, breathing hurried, the membrane of the nose and eyes red. Turning the horse short round, or hitting against the chest, back of the shoulder, will cause a kind of grunt.

Treatment.—Blanket warmly, and put in a comfortable stall, where there will be pure air, and give aconite, prepared as follows: Tinc. aconite, 1 oz.; water, 3 oz. Of this give from fifteen to thirty drops every twenty or thirty minutes, on the tongue, giving more or less according to the severity of the case. If the case is severe apply some strong stimulant to the legs and on each side of the body and breast, such as mustard, made into a paste and rubbed in thoroughly, or a liniment composed of aqua ammonia, reduced one-half with water; or any strong stimulating liniment should be applied. The aconite should be repeated every twenty or thirty minutes until relieved, lessening the dose both in proportion and frequency as the condition of the animal improves.

Note.—If you give a few doses of aconite about the time fever sets in, or before, the horse will be relieved next day.

INFLAMMATION OF THE LUNGS

is first noticeable by the horse having a severe chill or shivering fit. He refuses his food, hangs his head between the fore legs or upon the manger, will not move or lie down, breathing quick and short, panting like. The nostrils are expanded, the head thrown forward; the countenance expresses pain and great prostration. (See cut.) The pulse is some-

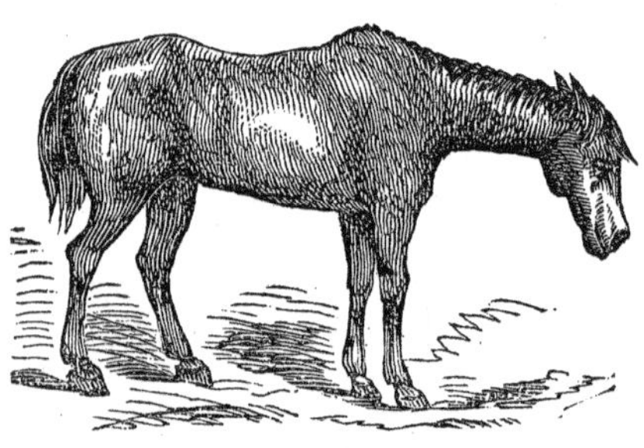

The Commencement of Inflammation of the Lungs.

times full and quick, but generally quick and weak, scarcely perceptible; the membrane of the nose and eyes bright red, tending to purple; ears and legs very cold; a choking noise sometimes coming from the throat.

Note.—In severe cases the horse may be very restless, lie down and get up very suddenly, resembling colic. Here the practitioner may be deceived if not careful to observe closely.

In some cases a little blood may be thrown from one or both nostrils. Extreme prostration and laborious breathing and bleeding from nostrils shows severe congestion of the lungs. In this case relief must be prompt, or the horse may die from suffocation.

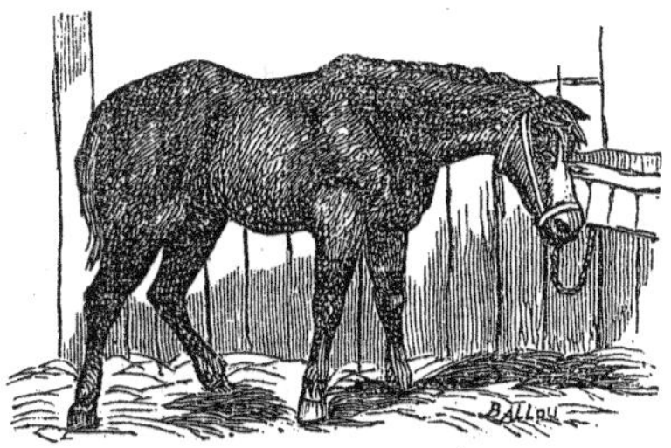

Congestion of the Lungs.

Treatment.—As the first object now is to reduce the congestion, it will be necessary to take from four to six quarts of blood from the neck vein. Stimulate the sides and legs as for pleurisy, and give aconite, prepared in the same manner, every ten minutes until the fever subsides, when small doses are to be repeated at intervals of a few hours as the case improves. Oil or physic must not be given in the treatment of any of the forms of inflammation of the lungs, as such so intensifies the inflammation as to often make the case terminate fatally.

In all ordinary cases of inflammation of the lungs all that is necessary to do is to put the horse in a well ventilated stall, blanket and give aconite. A few swallows of water should be given occasionally, and if the horse will drink, the medicine may be given in the water. Watch the pulse and the condition of the animal. In health the pulse is about 40 beats to the minute, regular and full. In inflammation of the lungs it may run up to 70 or even 80 beats, and so light as to be scarcely felt even by the touch of the experienced practitioner. Improvement will be denoted by the pulse becoming fuller and more regular, and the countenance will become more lively. I have known many cases to apparently resist treatment for days, the condition of the animal continuing about

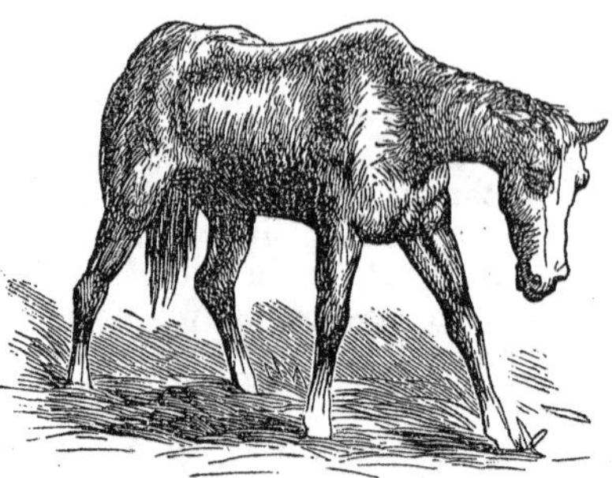

Position Assumed by a Horse During a Severe Attack of Inflammation of the Lungs.

the same, and then yield readily. Usually the improvement is marked from the start. Of course it is desirable, when the case is severe, to resort to active counter irritation, to excite the blood to the extremities. The mustard, ammonia or other stimulating preparations recommended should be used three or four times a day.

If the pulse is high and obstinate, and does not yield to the above treatment, alternate by giving *tincture veratrum*, in the proportion of about ten or fifteen drops in a little water on the tongue, repeated every thirty or forty minutes until there is a noticeable effect upon the pulse. It is also sometimes advisable to alternate with a few doses of belladonna, given in the same proportion.

It is hardly safe to recommend any complication of treatment that would possibly confuse or mislead. This is perhaps the safest and most practical treatment ever given to the public, and if used in a reasonable time, and with any degree of prudence, is almost sure to cure.

After improvement, diet should be low for some time—gruel and bran mashes, not much at a time; a few carrots or potatoes, and no oats or corn, and but little if any hay.

TYPHOID PNEUMONIA, OR A LOW TYPE OF INFLAMMATION OF THE LUNGS.

This disease sometimes assumes an epidemic form, and is both dangerous and treacherous if not anticipated and properly treated.

Though a common and fatal disease, it is not laid down in any veterinary works I have seen, and in consequence of ignorance of its nature and improper treatment, is very fatal.

Symptoms.—The horse is dull, off his feed, disinclination to move, pulse about 50, weak or low; will sometimes eat a little hay; will not lie down; not much cough; barely any discoloration of the membrane of the nose or eyes; urine scanty and high-colored; fæces hard and coated; after two or three days the membrane of the nose and eyes a little more discolored or red; pulse quicker; there is a discharge from one or both nostrils, usually one; the breathing is quicker; about the sixth or seventh day there is a large flow of urine, is more clear and watery in appearance; the legs swell and there is a watery secretion under the belly, after or during which there may be lameness, usually in one of the fore legs, which may soon change to the other.

The main point in treating the disease is to keep the fever down without lowering the strength. Bleeding or physic must not on any account be resorted to. Give aconite as for the other cases, observing the same care in blanketing and putting in a clean, well ventilated stall. Nurse and tempt the appetite by giving warm gruel and such mild delicacies as the horse will eat. If the pulse is above seventy, give more aconite; if below that, less. This fever will run its course in about seven or eight days. Nurse carefully; the animal will show great prostration, and recuperates slowly, and must not be put to work until fully recovered. Do not give any physic or attempt to bleed. A fatal result will almost surely follow depletion. On the contrary, it is often necessary in critical cases, where the system is low and the strength is reduced, to give tonics. The safest and best course for the reader to pursue is to keep and build up the strength by careful nursing. Give all the feed, at all times, the horse will eat. It is highly important to keep the appetite good and keep the strength up.

Catarrh, or Cold.

Cold is of common occurrence, and may lead to very serious consequences if neglected. If looked to in time, with a little rest and nursing, the system will soon resume its normal condition.

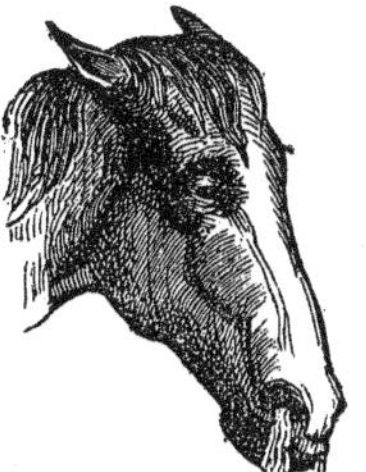

Effect of a Cold.

The usual symptoms are, a little increase of pulse, a slight discharge from the nose and eyes, the hair roughed, not much appetite, and some cough, which is sometimes severe.

Blanket warmly, give aconite as for

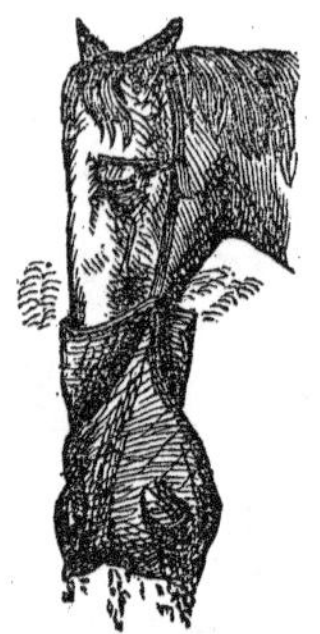

Steaming the Nose of a Horse having Cold.

fever. Nurse by giving bran mashes, &c. If the case is serious it may run into general inflammation of the air passages, as bronchitis or laryngitis. Would aim to keep up the strength, giving fever medicine, alternating with belladonna. Put on a bag, made of coarse, loose cloth, into which put some bran on which throw an ounce or two of turpentine. Now pour on some hot water. Hang the bag on the head, same as in cut, being careful not to have it so tight around the nose as to heat or scald and be oppressive. A few repetitions of this will cause the nose to run freely. Rest and care will usually do the rest.

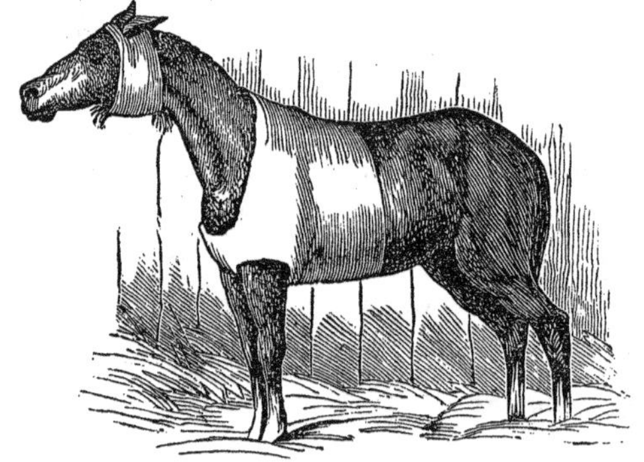

If there is obstinate inflammation of the throat and air passages, any good liniment may be applied around the chest and throat and bandaged, as shown in the cut. The object is to stimulate the surface, and this would be an easy, practical way of doing it.

Strangles.

This is another form of sore-throat, familiar to every one. Its design seems to be to throw some poisonous matter from the system, and the object should be to keep the strength of the animal up and hasten suppuration.

The horse is out of sorts; the neck becomes sore and stiff; an enlargement appears which is first hard and tender; there is some discharge from the nose. The case usually grows worse, if very severe, often threatening to cause suffocation; horse unable to eat or drink but little, and strength is lost rapidly.

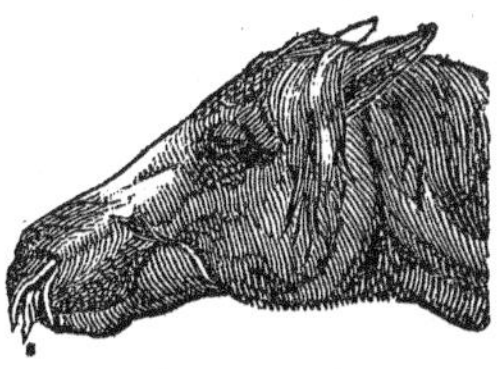

Strangles.

Use freely a poultice made of wheat bran and warm vinegar, changing as often as the poultice becomes dry, using the eight-tailed bandage, until the enlargement becomes soft and can be opened, when relief will be prompt. Or the following treatment may be adopted, which is similar, and if the alteration is not good, is preferable: Take spirits of turpentine, two parts; spirits of camphor, one part; laudanum, one part. Put this on the neck with a brush, if convenient, or any way to apply it without exciting pain, three or four times a day until soreness is caused. After each application have ready three or four pieces of flannel, which should be a good thick article;

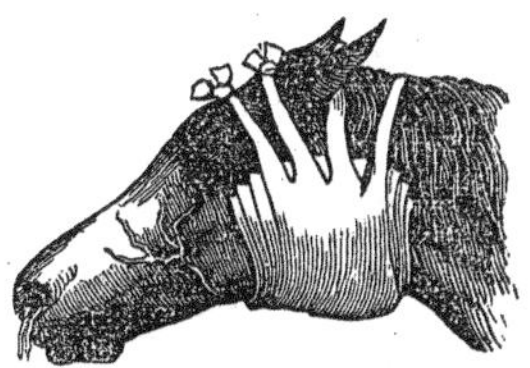

Applying an Eight-Tailed Bandage in Strangles.

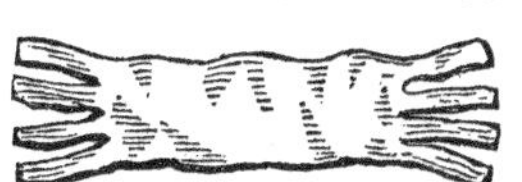

Eight-Tailed Bandage.

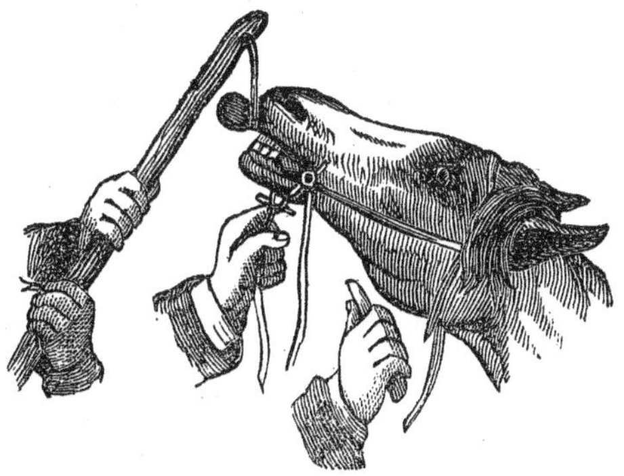

Opening the Abscess in Strangles.

put these over the parts and bind on with the eight-tailed bandage. When the tumor points, open it, and be sure that the matter has a thorough outlet. Sometimes the inflammation is so deep as to cause serious soreness and swelling of the throat. In this case the horse must be nursed carefully by feeding with warm gruel; the drink should be warm; grass or anything that will tempt the appetite should be given. Physic must not be given.

Inflammation of the Bowels.

This disease is generally caused by constipation of the bowels, hard driving, over-purging or looseness of bowels, or drinking cold water when warm. Constipation is, however, the principal cause of the disease, and when this is the case, the first and most important condition of relief is to get an action of the bowels.

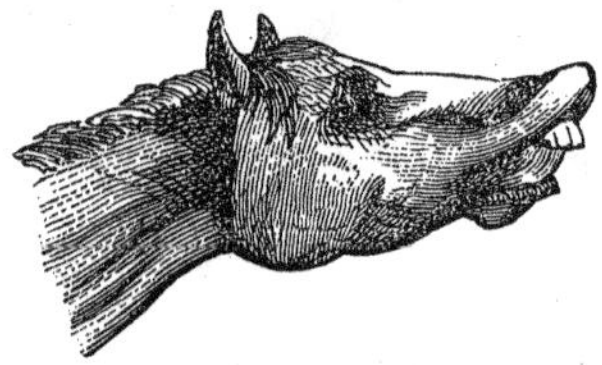

Symptoms of Intestinal and Abdominal Irritation, as Shown in Inflammation of the Bowels.

Symptoms.—For the first few hours the horse is uneasy, paws, looks around at the side, the pulse is slightly accelerated and wiry. As the disease advances the intermissions between the attack become less, pulse quicker, running from seventy to eighty beats in a minute, in some instances even faster; lies down and gets up, shows much pain, no swelling of sides. Now begins to exhibit fever, bowels constipated, urine highly colored and scanty.

Remedy.—Give a quart of raw linseed oil.

Note.—If constipation is very great, add from four to six drops of croton oil.

If scours or over-purging, give an ounce and a half of the tincture of opium with six ounces of water. But in order to suppress the inflammation it is necessary to bleed immediately from the neck vein from six to ten quarts of blood, according to the strength and size of the animal. In extreme cases bleeding may be repeated to the extent of four to six quarts in three or four hours. If much pain exists in constipation, give from one to three ounces tincture asafœtida. Feed lightly for a week at least, giving gruel, roots, grass and bran mashes, and keep quiet. No exercise for several days if there is danger of a relapse.

Inflammation of the Kidneys.

Inflammation of the kidneys is generally caused by hard work, by slipping, throwing the hind parts so suddenly under the belly as to produce undue tension of the lumbar vertebræ, or from sudden colds by being exposed to rain and cold, the eating of musty hay or oats, or unhealthy food of any kind. Too powerful or too often repeated diuretics produce inflammation of the kidneys, or a degree of irritation and weakness of them that disposes to inflammation, from causes that would otherwise have no injurious effect.

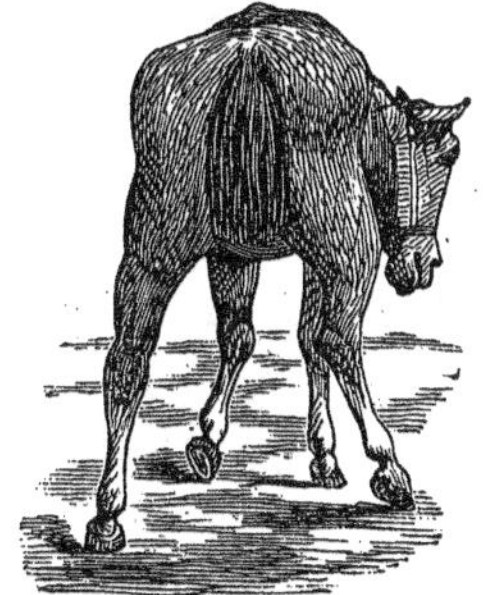

Appearance of a Horse Suffering from Diseases of the Urinary Organs.

Symptoms.—Less or more fever of the system generally, and unwillingness to move, particularly the hind legs, dung hard and coated, very sensitive to pressure on the spine. The horse looks anxiously round at his flanks, stands with his hind legs wide apart, straddles as he walks, shows pain in turning; the urine is voided in small quantities, and is usually high colored, sometimes bloody; the attempt to urinate becomes more frequent, and the quantity voided smaller, until the animal strains violently, without being able to pass any or but very little urine. The pulse is quick and hard, full in the early stage of the disease, but rapidly becoming small, though not losing its character of hardness. Introduce the hand into the rectum. If the bladder is found full and hard under the rectum, there is inflammation of the neck of the bladder. If the bladder is empty, yet on the portion of the intestines immediately over it there is more than natural heat and tenderness, there is inflammation of the body of the bladder. If the bladder is empty and there is

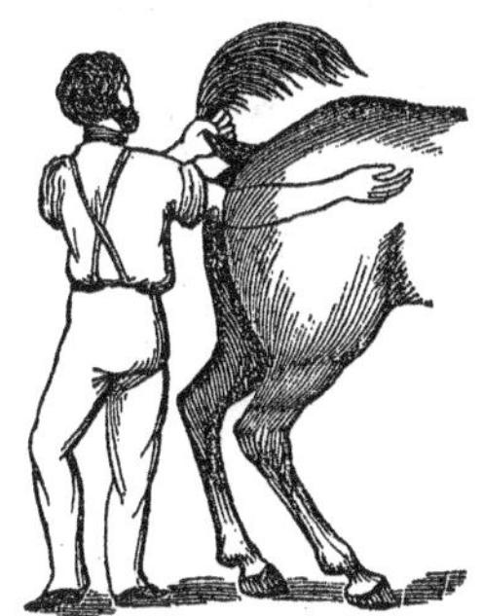

Test for Inflammation of the Kidneys.

no increased tenderness and heat, there is inflammation of the kidneys.

Treatment.—If the pulse is high, about sixty, take five or six quarts of blood and give a fever ball; to be repeated in three hours if not better. Fever ball: 4 drams Barbadoes aloes, 1 dram tartar emetic, 2 drams ginger, calomel about the size of a bean, molasses sufficient to make into a ball. Counter irritation must next be excited over the seat of the disease. The loins should be fomented with hot water or covered with mustard poultice, or, better, heat a peck of salt in an oven, place it in a bag, and put it over the part affected. If the case is severe and protracted, a sharp blister may be used. *No diuretics are to be given, as they would simply aggravate*, and make the disease worse. After the bowels are open, give aconite, and treat as for fever. After recovery the horse should be kept very quiet for a month, and if in season, turned out to grass. If in winter, feed with light mashy diet; exercise lightly by leading, if the animal be valuable and it is desired to aid recovery by extra care.

Inflammation of the Bladder.

Symptoms almost the same as those of inflammation of the kidneys. Frequent voiding of urine in small quantities, quick pulse, looks frequently at flanks, paws violently, tender when pressed upon under the flanks.

Here the principal object is to lower inflammation and relax the muscular contraction of the neck of the bladder. Bleed largely, almost to fainting; give physic as for inflammation of the kidneys, or a quart of linseed oil. A dram of powdered opium, made into a ball, or given in drink, every two or three hours, and blister over the loins. Give aconite, as for inflammation of the kidneys.

Inflammation of the Brain, or Staggers,

Is first noticeable by dullness or sleepiness of the eyes, an unwillingness to move, general heaviness of the system. This disease is frequently called *megrims, fits and mad staggers;* but in part only one disease, according to the extent of such disease as the animal may be affected with.

In my opinion, there is but one cause for staggers, that is, an undue flow of blood to the brain, which rarely or never occurs in any animals except those in a plethoric (fat) condition.

Some writers and practitioners assert that there is a disease known as stomach staggers. I have never seèn a case where it was necessary to treat the stomach, but always direct attention to the brain, as being the seat of this disease, which may be properly called *head staggers.*

In cases of megrims or fits it is merely a lesser attack, or pressure of the blood-vessels on the brain, and *mad staggers* is a greater pressure of the same vessels on the same part. The brain is divided into two parts, namely, cerebrum and cerebellum, which occupy a horny box in the head. The blood-vessels passing over the brain and coming in contact with the skull, become distended by an increased quantity of blood, and produce the feeling, which is thus exhibited.

There is but one cure for this disease, and that is, remove the cause. Bleed largely from the neck—ten, twelve or fourteen quarts, or until the symptoms of fainting. After the horse is convalescent a sharp dose of physic should be given to regulate the bowels. I would advise owners of such horses to dispose of them. Once taken with the disease, they are subject to a repetition of the attack when the blood-vessels become filled again.

Note.—Small doses of aconite (of the quantity for fever) may be given three or four times a day as a good preventive. Turning horses to pasture that may be liable to this disease will prove both injurious and dangerous.

Founder, (Laminitis.)

There are two stages of this disease, acute and chronic. The first produces a high state of excitement and inflammation of the sensible laminæ of the foot. The second, a morbid or insensible feeling of the parts generally. The first is invariably cured if properly treated. The second is not curable, but may be palliated to a limited extent. Acute founder is easily detected. The animal invariably extends the fore feet as far forward as he can, and brings the hind ones in the same position under him. There is so much pain in the fore feet that he endeavors to throw his weight on the hind ones. (See cut.) The common causes of founder are exposing the animal when warm to sudden changes, usually produced by the following means, namely: Standing in cold air when warm, after being driven, driving through a river while warm, or giving cold water to drink while warm, washing the feet when warm and neglecting to dry them, &c. It is generally supposed that feeding a horse while warm will produce founder. This is an error, unless it is such food as will chill the system, which may be done by giving a large quantity of cold wet mixed feed, whereby the circulation would be checked, as before explained.

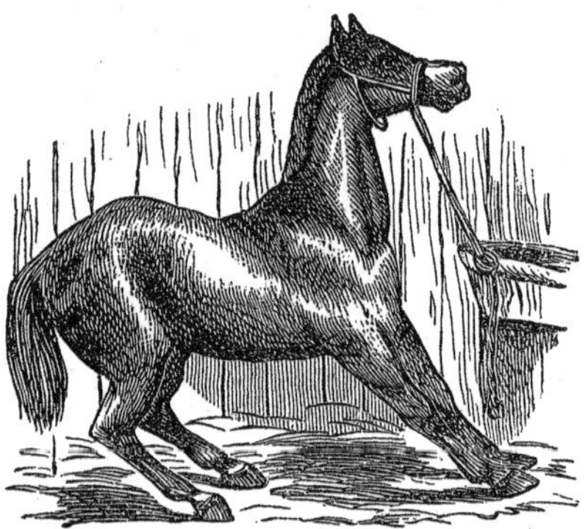

The Horse as he Appears when Suffering from Inflammation in the Feet, or Founder.

To come right to the point, founder is simply inflammation in the feet, whatever of general disturbance of the system is caused by the pain and soreness in them, and the correct principle of cure is to lower and remove this inflammation before change of structure or sloughing can take place.

Treatment.—As soon as the disease has developed itself, bleed from the neck, according to the size and condition of the animal—from six to twelve quarts. Then give a sharp cathartic ball—7 drams aloes, 4 drams bar soap, 1 dram ginger. Make into a ball and give immediately. After the fore shoes have been removed, poultice thoroughly with bran wet with cold water. This poultice may, while on the feet, be kept wet by dipping the poulticed foot into a pail of cold water, or pouring some on. This poulticing should be kept up from four to five days, when the shoes may be tacked on, and the animal exercised a little. Cloths wet with cold water should be tied around the coronet and the soles stuffed for a week or two. The horse should have tepid water to drink and warm bran mashes during the operation of the medicine. If the disease should be stubborn, which is rarely the case, a second ball may be given after an interval of five days.

Nothing can be done for a sub-acute founder, or case badly treated. If the sole is broken down do not pare the sole. Fit the shoe so as not to press on the sole. Stuff the whole bottom with oakum and tar, and apply leather over. Put on the shoe carefully. Cure is impossible. If warm fomentations are used, instead of cold, a relaxation of the sensible laminæ on the wall of the foot is liable to take place. This throws the entire weight on the sole, through the os pedis, forcing it through at the toe.

There are but few who will attempt to bleed as directed, and fewer still who will give a ball, (special directions for doing which will be found in another chapter.) If you cannot bleed or physic as directed, bleed from the toes, if you can, standing the fore feet in moderately warm water while doing so, and give aconite as for inflammation of the lungs. Keep the feet wet by poulticing or standing in cold watei until relieved. Use cloths and stuff as before directed.

This treatment even will cure, but the first treatment given affords prompt relief. No dependence can be placed upon pretended *sure cure* for founder. The treatment here given is specific, and can be relied upon.

Heaves, or Broken Wind.

Heaves produces increased action of the flanks. The inspiration is natural, but the expiration requires two motions to expel the air. There is always a short cough, or grunt, and at the same time expels wind while coughing. Heaves are never found in the racing stable, where horses are properly fed. They are always found among cart or team horses, where the owners suppose they must feed a large quantity of coarse food or hay.

The seat of the disease is located in the air cells of the lungs, causing enlargement and sometimes a rupture of these cells. This disease is often produced by forcing too large a quantity of food into the stomach and bowels, and the greedy animal, not being even then satisfied, eats the bedding.

He is then taken out and worked or driven hard, the bowels and stomach pressing on the diaphram, thereby not allowing the lungs to expand by being filled with air, and by this increased pressure the air cells are enlarged or ruptured, and the horse is said to have the heaves. Much has been said by different authors regarding the curability of heaves. Some advocate one means and some another, among which is that of feeding on Western plains, or prairie grass, or feeding prairie hay, which is said to contain resin weed, that will effect a cure. Prairie hay is only a palliative, affording relief so long only as used. Prairie hay or grass is more laxative than timothy hay, and the animal cannot eat half as much in a given time of the former as of the latter, consequently it not only promotes a condition favorable to respiration, by stimulating the bowels, but does not cause that pressure upon the lungs that the timothy in consequence does. While prairie hay has a decidedly beneficial effect in alleviating heaves, there are several other kinds of food equally as good, or better, than prairie hay or grass. One is, cornstalk fodder. As it is the amount of saccharine matter that food contains which makes it valuable, and the less compass it occupies in the bowels the better, we must arrive at this conclusion, and experience proves it to be correct. One quart of oats is equal to an armful of hay, and three pounds of corn leaves contain more sugar than six times the bulk of hay. The cause, the cure and treatment is marked in these words, that heaves is produced by pressure on the diaphram, by too much food in the stomach and bowels, and is cured by lessening the quantity of a better quality of food, to occupy the same space. If horses are turned out to grass, after a few days heaves will generally disappear, from the fact that the bowels are generally relaxed by taking exercise and having pure air.

The only treatment which will prove in any degree effective is as follows: first give one of the following balls: Ginger, powdered, ½ oz.; capsicum, ¼ oz. Form a ball. This ball to be given three nights in succession; then omit two or three nights, and one or two balls may be given again in succession; or eight or ten drops of tincture of phosphorus may be given in drink several times a day for eight or ten days. The horse should have regular exercise, be watered often, (small quantities at a time,) and have straw instead of hay to eat, (corn fodder would be much better.) Under this treatment heaves will disappear.

FAVORITE REMEDIES OF GREAT VALUE FOR HEAVES.

1. Spanish brown, 2 oz.; tartar emetic, 2 oz.; resin, 4 oz.; ginger, 2 oz. Mix and give two teaspoonfuls twice a day in the feed.

2. Vegetable tar, in mass, ½ oz.; gum camphor, ½ oz.; tartar emetic, 1 dram. Form into a ball, one of which is to be given once a day. If proper attention is given to feeding, this will cure the heaves in three days, unless very bad.

3. The following prescription is one of the very best remedies known for heaves, and will in many cases cure: Take indigo, 1 oz.; saltpeter, 1 oz.; rain water, 1 gallon; mix and give a pint twice a day in the feed.

Tetanus, or Locked Jaw.

This disease is wholly of a nervous character. A description of the symptoms is scarcely necessary, but in the first stage there is a disinclination to move; then the tail becomes erect and quivers, the ears set back, and the conjunctina (hair) is thrown over the pupils of the eye, and the head is elevated.

As the disease advances the muscles all over the neck and body become stiff and rigid, and the legs have the appearance of a four-footed stool. The animal has little or no power to move.

For the first few days the teeth remain apart, but as the disease advances the muscles of the jaw become so contracted as to bring them close together. Hence the name of locked jaw.

The causes of this disease are numerous, but it is generally produced from a wounded nerve or bunch of nerves, pricking the tail, and very often from docking, punctured wounds in the feet from glass or nails, and sometimes from severe exposure to cold, and I have known one case to occur from fright. As to the pulse, it is almost normal for the first few days. As the disease advances the pulse quickens, and the animal is compelled to stand on his legs until death, if it terminates fatally. If favorably, a relaxation of the muscles begins from the fifth to the seventh day. This disease is more common in the extreme South than in the North.

Treatment.—First, as the disease is of a nervous character, quietness is of the greatest importance. The animal should be put into an isolated place or box, by himself, and the cause of the disease found. If from docking, the next joint should be taken off the tail. If from a wound in the foot, the wound should be opened up and made new, and an application of digestive ointment inserted, so as to produce a healthy flow of matter. When the irritation has ceased from the wound, a pail of gruel should be placed before him, in which is mixed half an ounce of tartar emetic. This medicine should be given daily, and the spine rubbed well with a strong liniment, composed of one part of aqua ammonia and two parts of sweet oil. This embrocation should be employed daily until the back becomes sore.

Tetanus never arises from a wound until about the period that it may be considered healed. Bleeding about four quarts daily for four or five days has cured several bad cases. Think if the bowels can be regulated, quietness has more to do in producing a cure than all other remedies.

Spavin and Ringbone.

There are two kinds of bone spavin, namely: Jack and ocult, or consolidated joint. The first is located at the upper portion of the metatarsal bone at its juncture with the cuboid bones. The second is usually located higher up and more on the inside of the astragalus bone at its junction with the cuboid bones.

Spavins of either of the above classes have the same origin and same causes, namely, inflammation of the cartilage of the joint in the first instance, and extending to ulceration of the bone, consequently bony matter is thrown out, uniting more or less of the bone of the hock and excess of matter and ulceration of the bones from the enlargement.

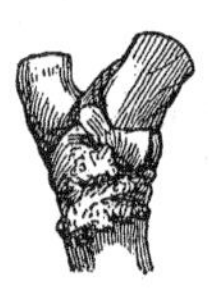

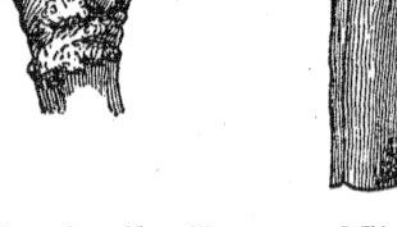

Showing the Changes of Structure Caused.

The causes of spavin are numerous, but principally of one class, such as sprains, hard work, blows, and, in fact, any cause exciting inflammation of this part. But a common cause and a great fault lies in the breeders of horses, as very often the colt is bred from spavin sire or dam, or both, and the colt is certain to inherit the same predisposition.

The symptoms at the commencement are treacherous. Very often horses are treated for hip lameness, before any enlargement makes its appearance. The horse, at first, is very lame while laboring under acute inflammation of the hock joint. He will not wear out of the lameness as he does in the more advanced stage of the disease. The tumor generally makes its appearance from the fifth to the eighth week. Sometimes, however, the lameness is very gradual—scarcely perceptible at first—getting worse until there is marked lameness at starting, which will soon wear off as the horse warms up.

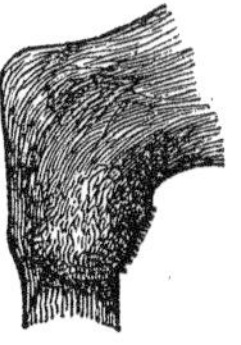
Bone Spavin.

The method of curing is varied as there are hundreds of different remedies and applications. Some men go so far as to pretend they can remove spavins. To a skillful practitioner this is absurd. It will be seen that if such quacks *can* remove the external tumor, they *can not* separate the bones which are united, and horses may be spavined without any visible enlargement.

I can simplify all this to gentlemen interested, by illustrating what I mean, by my specimens, a good collection of which I carry for the purpose. Sublimates, muriatic and sulphuric, and nitric acids form the basis of the different ointments that are applied to remove this formidable disease. They always make a bad sore and blemish the animal for life.

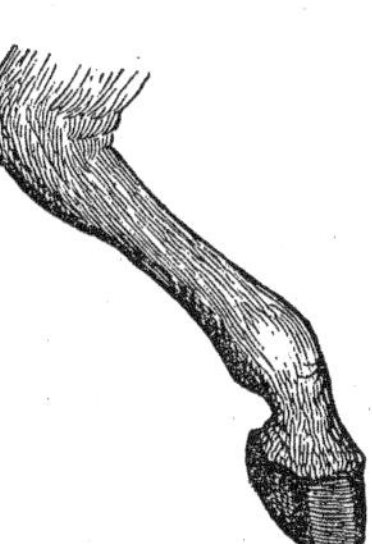
Natural Action.

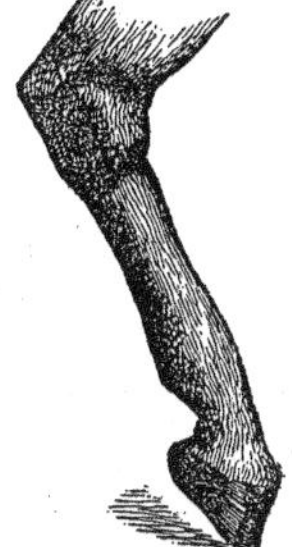
Effect of Bad Spavin —Leg not Brought Forward.

The only reasonable treatment for bone spavin is counter irritation and rest. If there is heat during the first few days, apply cooling applications, such as an ounce of sugar of lead to half a pail of ice water. Keep the leg wet for about two weeks, when it may pass off. A dose of physic should be given. If this stage has passed, repeated blistering with a preparation of iodine or cantharidine will be necessary; but much better would be the actual cautery in an operator's hands. Clip the hair closely over a large surface four or five inches above and below the enlargement, and then out to the middle of the back and fore parts of the leg. Any of the strong blisters recommended for spavins, for which formulas are given in another chapter, are to be used. If a blister, rub it in well with the hand for ten minutes or more. In two days put on some grease. When the inflammation goes down, wash with warm water and castile soap, and when dry put on more blister, and so repeat, keeping up just as much irritation as you can without destroying the hair. In the mean time, the horse must be kept in a comfortable stall, for one of the conditions of cure is rest. Keep up the inflammation in this way for four or five weeks, after which give a run to grass. It is sometimes necessary to blister lightly, if the lameness does not disappear in six or eight weeks, which may be repeated a few times, with iodine ointment in the proportion of one part of iodine to two of lard.

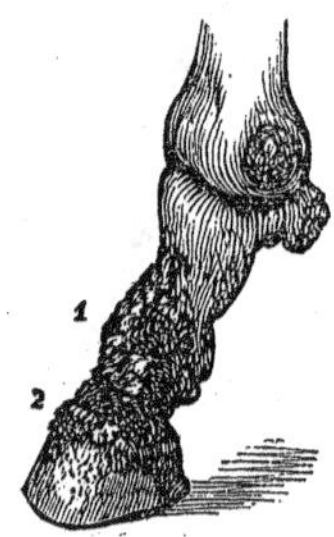

Ringbone.

Work should be light, if any, within three months. This treatment will usually cure without leaving a blemish.

Treat ringbones on the same principle. Trim off the hair and blister in the same manner, observing the same condition of rest. As regards taking off the enlargement, this treatment is as effectual towards that end as can be used.

Several of the very best recipes for the cure of spavins and ringbones will be found in another chapter.

BLOOD SPAVIN, THOROUGH PIN,

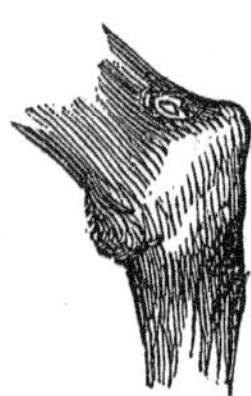
Thorough Pin.

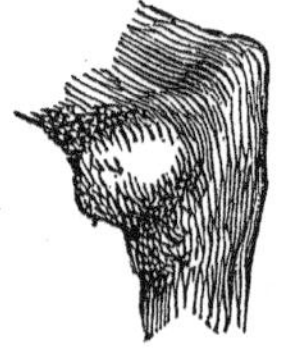
Bog, or Blood Spavin.

Soft enlargements upon the hock. Treatment the same. If not of long standing, the following will be found very effective, though simple: Rub on soft soap at night, and wash off in the morning, repeating until cured. Two or three applications will cure, if recently caused. If of long duration, blister two or three times, clipping the hair as for spavin. If the enlargement is very great and of long standing, it is difficult to do much.

SPRAIN OF THE BACK SINEWS.

The animal becomes suddenly lame, and by use grows worse. Pass the fingers down on each of the tendons back of the knee. A little enlargement, if there, with considerable inflammation, will be discovered. Use cooling astringent liniment until the acute stage passes off. If not better then, blister, observing to give the animal rest. It is sometimes very obstinate.

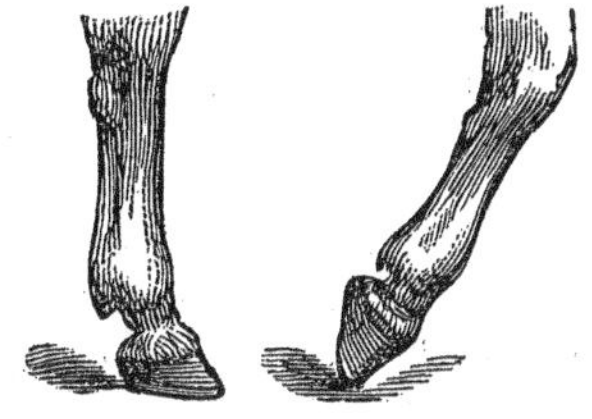

Enlargement Caused by Sprain of the Tendons.

SPLINTS.

This is an enlargement between the cannon and splint bones, showing itself on the inside of the fore leg. The same treatment as for spavin.

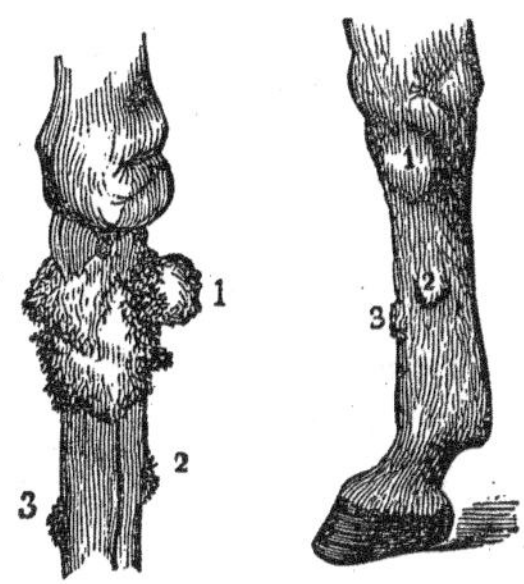

Changes that may be Produced. Splint.

CURB.

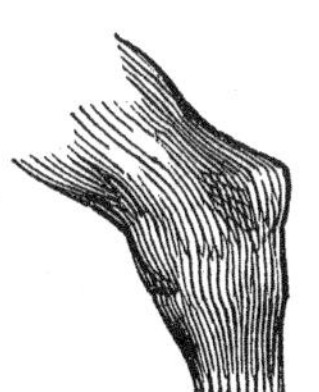

Clean Hock.

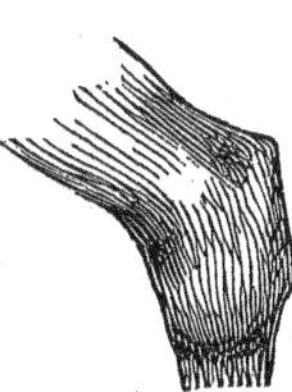

Curb.

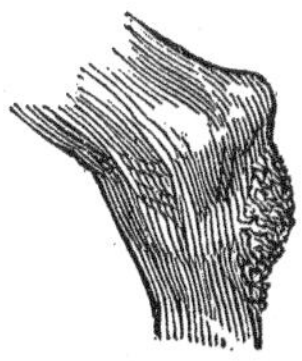

Curb.

This is an enlargement of the integument, and in some cases of bony deposit, usually caused by a strain. It is situated on the back part of the hock, just below the cap. Same treatment as for spavin.

Coffin Joint Lameness

Is often mistaken by those who are not capable of locating the diseases of horses' feet to be lameness of the shoulder, from the fact that generally after the shoe is removed, and no external injury is discovered in the foot, some distant part is selected as the location of the disease. Navicular disease is dangerous and treacherous in its progress and development. It is commonly caused by violent sprains of the navicular joint, although sometimes, and, in fact, very often, may be induced by a contusion of the frog; and again, there is a disposition to have this disease from hereditary causes.

The coffin joint is composed of three bones: the os pedis, the navicular and small pastern bones. The navicular bone answers the purpose of a support in allowing great elasticity of motion. The flexor tendon inserts itself into the os pedis, and passes immediately over the navicular bone, so that at each step the navicular bone is thrown upon one part of the os pedis and small pastern at the same time. It will be seen that in all cases of lameness of this joint, as well as in any other joint lameness, that the cartilage of the bones is inflamed, and as the disease progresses ulceration takes place, and consequently ancholosis. It is almost striving against hope to be able to explain to the general reader the symptoms to enable ability to locate the disease with any degree of certainty. Corns or bruises of the sole, contraction, or almost any cause exciting inflammation in the foot, may cause similar lameness, and to an ordinary observer there cannot be that fine judgment necessary to trace from certain peculiarities the location of the trouble.

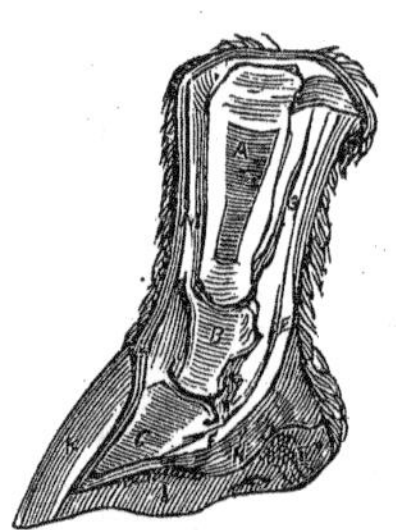

Section of the Parts Entering into the Composition of the Foot, and the Fetlock and Pastern Joints.

a Os suffraginis. *b* Os coronæ. *c* Os pedis. *d* Os naviculare. *e e* The perforans and perforatus tendons. *g* Inferior sesamoideal ligament. *h* Cleft of frog. *i* Side of frog cleft. *j* Sole. *k* Crust. *l* Coronary substance.

Horses having navicular disease invariably travel more on the toe than on the heel, consequently the shoe is always worn more at the toe than at the heel. The hoof rarely or never is malformed, but the disease commonly occurs in healthy looking feet contraction of one or both heels, which will in many cases interfere with the outer cartilage of the joint. In cases of long standing the frog appears to recede, and does not have a natural appearance. If the horse is taken suddenly lame, sometimes scarcely putting the foot down, and only presses upon the toe, feel of the foot carefully. If there is heat around the top of the hoof and tenderness—even a little at the heel—there is probably strain of the coffin joint. In incipent cases (first stages) there is fever and tenderness to motion of the joint, which is noticeable by catching the foot in one hand, the ankle in the other, and twisting a little. The animal will show pain and resist.

As to treatment, in the first stage, the shoe should be removed, and have the toe of the shoe hammered down. The heels should be raised, and applied again so as to remove all pressure from the frog, and a cloth or rug saturated with cold water applied to the coronet. The bottom of the foot should be stuffed with oil meal or some adhesive substance. If this is done for a few days, with rest, the first attack will generally pass off.

In the more advanced stage of this disease it will require thorough treatment. The shoe should be formed and applied as before, and a severe blistering applied to the coronet, which should be continued for from one to three weeks, with rest. At a still more advanced stage the frog seaton may be used, but this must be done by an experienced practitioner.

In all cases of this disease the animal will require considerable rest.

I would here remark that in an advanced stage of the disease the horse is a little lame, sometimes worse, at others better; rough road and down hill worse; is no worse to be at work; usually no apparent change in the hoof; will go better when the heels are raised by using high-heeled shoes; worse by bringing heels to the ground.

Sweeny.

This is an affection of the muscles of the upper part of the shoulder. It is characterized by a shrinking of the shoulder, with lameness. It is called atrophy, or wasting away of the muscles of the upper part of the shoulder. The cause of sweeny is dependent upon some other difficulty. Contraction, corns, etc., or any cause preventing a proper use of the limb.

Examine the foot carefully, discover the cause, and, if possible, remove it. Next, take oil of spike, 2 oz.; oil of organum, 2 oz.; aqua ammonia, 2 oz.; spirits of turpentine, 2 oz.; sweet oil, 2 oz.; alcohol, 2 oz.; mix. This is to be applied freely to the shrunken parts and well rubbed in every other day. Four or five applications will cure.

The usual method of cure is by a seaton. The needle is passed through the skin at the upper border of the shrunken part and passed down under the skin and out at the lower border. The tape is then drawn through and the ends are knotted together. The tape should be smeared with Venice turpentine or a little blistering ointment, or fifteen or twenty drops of tincture of Spanish flies may be dropped into the opening. The seaton should be washed every day. In fifteen or twenty days the seaton can be taken out, and the sweeny will be cured.

Retention of Urine.

The most common cause is keeping the animal at work, not giving time to urinate, and a spasm of the neck of the bladder or gravelly concretions; any cause of irritation may cause spasm. Symptoms are the same as in inflammation of the kidneys, except standing very wide behind, and when walking, a straddling gait resembling a cow with a very full bag.

The most prompt treatment is to use the catheter, and scarcely anything more is necessary. But if one is not obtainable, bleed freely and give a strong opiate. 3 oz. tinc. opium, in half pint of water.

Scours or Purging.

This disease is generally produced by two causes: change of food or water, or unhealthy food, and sometimes through nervous excitement.

Cure.—Neutralize the acids in the bowels by giving an ounce and a half of prepared chalk and a dram and a half of prepared catechu, mixed in a pint of water. Give once or twice a day until purging ceases. Keep the animal without exercise, and do not give much water to drink.

The treatment given in the following pages will be found very valuable, as it is written up in plain language, and the very best treatment given. There are single remedies given here worth far more than the cost of the book.

Spasmodic Action of the Diaphragm, (Thumps,)

Is caused by severe and long-continued driving and hard work. Horses of a nervous temperament having too much cold water given to drink on a cold morning, nervous irritation, or excitement from any cause, may excite this trouble.

Symptoms.—A sudden jerking or twitching of the muscles of the sides and flanks; pulse wiry, quick and low, more or less fever; extremities natural.

Cure.—This disease being of a purely spasmodic character, but in this case wholly of a nervous nature, bleeding must be omitted, and must be treated wholly by giving spasmodic remedies. Give asafœtida, in a dose of from 1 to 3 ounces of the tincture, mixed in a half pint of water. Given as a drench will stop it almost instantly.

If necessary, the medicine may be repeated in two hours. Keep the horse well clothed, and keep all exciting causes away from him. The bowels should be kept loose and regular, by giving bran mashes and moderate exercise.

Worms.

The symptoms of worms are debility, feebleness, sluggish movements, emaciation, staring coat, hide bound, skin covered with blotches, irregular and capricious appetite, tucked up belly, pallid appearance of the lining membrane of the lip, badly digested fæces, rubs the tail, and where fundament worms exist a whitish substance will be found about the fundament.

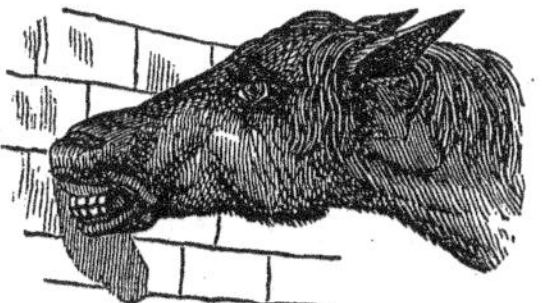

Symptoms of Worms.

Give of calomel, 3 drams; tartar emetic, 1 dram. Mix and divide into three powders; one to be given at night for three successive nights. To be followed, in twenty-four hours, with a good purging ball.

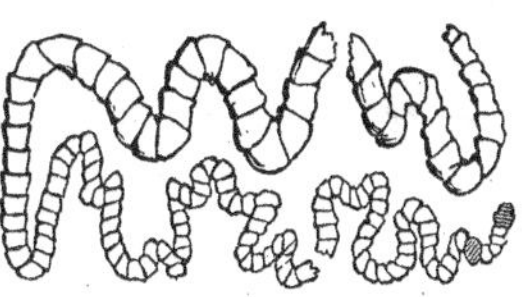

Tænia, or Tape Worm.

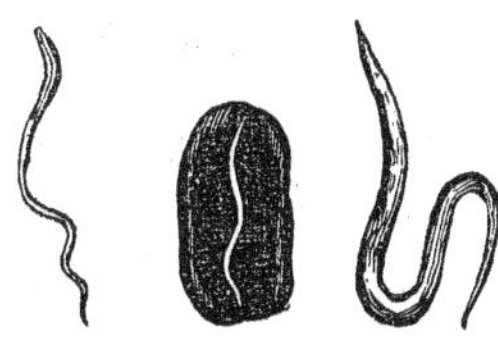

Different Kinds of Worms.

Bleeding.

For general bleeding the jugular vein is selected. The horse is blindfolded, or his head turned away; the hair is smoothed along the course of the vein with a moistened

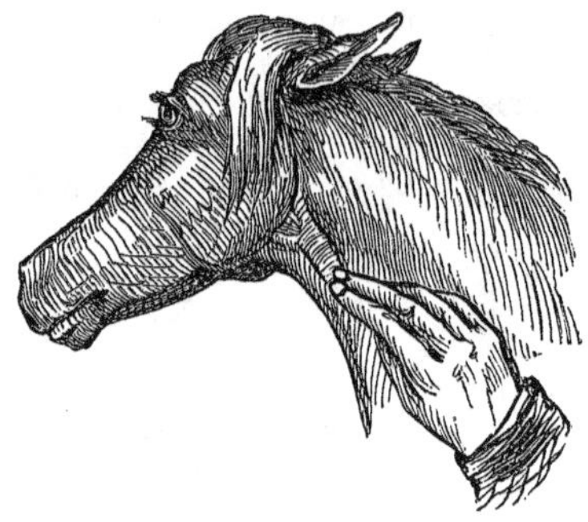

Raising the Vein.

finger, then, with the third and little fingers of the left hand, which holds the fleam, pressure is made on the vein sufficiently to bring it into view, but not to swell it too much. The point to be selected is about two inches below the union of the

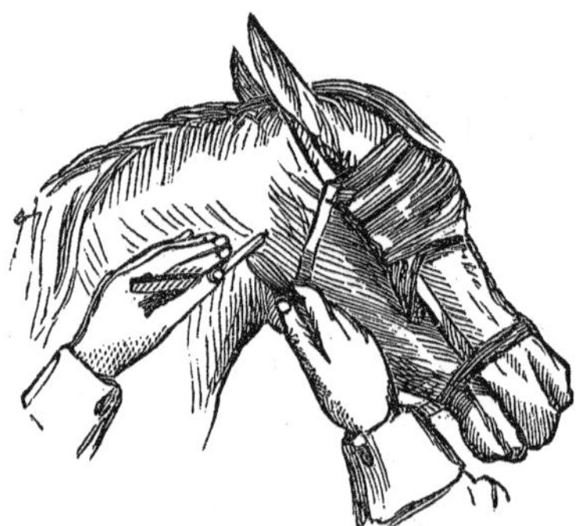

Bleeding from the Neck Vein.

jugular vein at the angle of the jaw. (See cut.) The fleam is put in a direct line with the vein at the center, when it is to be hit sharply with a stick. See that the fleam is large, sharp and clean, for if rusty or dull, inflammation of the vein might result. It is of great importance that the blood be drawn quickly. When sufficient blood has been taken, the edges of the wound should be brought closely together, and kept together by a small sharp pin being passed through them. Around this a little tow or a few hairs from the mane of the horse should be wrapped, so as to cover the whole of the incision, and the head of the horse should be tied up for several hours, to prevent his rubbing the part against the manger. When the bleeding is to be repeated, if more than three or four hours have elapsed, it will be more prudent to make a fresh incision, rather than to open the old wound.

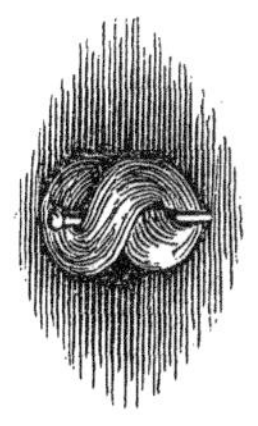

A pin is first stuck through the lips of the wound; a portion of tow, thread or hair is then wrapped round the pin.

Physicing.

It is always best, if possible, to prepare the horse for physic by giving a bran mash twenty-four hours previously, as the medicine will act more favorably and there is less danger of superpurgation. Five drams of aloes (Barbadoes aloes are always used for horses) will act as forcibly after a mash as seven without. Again, the quantity of physic should be adapted to age and size. The rule is to give one dram for each year up to seven. Eight drams is the largest given at one dose.

Physic Ball: Barbadoes aloes, pulverized, 7 drams; bar soap, 4 drams; ginger, 1 dram. The usual way is to mix the ingredients in this proportion, then reduce to the weight intended and give.

One ounce of tartar emetic is used by some practitioners for physic. It is more easily given.

For Alterative Balls simply give from one to two or three ounces of mass, as above prepared, two or three times a week, for a week or two.

For Worms: Give 4 drams aloes, 1 dram tartar emetic, 2 drams ginger, about the size of a bean of calomel, and molasses enough to make into a ball. To be given every morning for three days.

Condition Powders: Sulphur, 2 lbs.; fenugreek, 4 lbs.; cream tartar, 1 lb.; liquorice, 1 lb.; niter, 1 lb.; black antimony, ½ lb.; gentian, ¼ lb.; aniseed, ¼ lb.; common salt, 1 lb. Dose—One ounce daily, for two or three weeks.

CUTS OR WOUNDS—REMEDIES FOR.

If the cut or wound is very bad, trim the hair off close around the edges, and wash out carefully with warm water and castile soap. The object next is to produce a granulating process. There is hardly any use in sewing up cuts, as the stitches will sluff out.

Simple tincture of marigold, called callendula, has the best healing action of anything I have used. It will heal by first intention, and if a contused wound lowers inflammation and soreness. For man it is unrivalled, and I have found it equally good for horse flesh.

A fine healing lotion is: Tincture myrrh, 1 oz.; tincture aloes, 2 oz.; water, ½ pint. Mix, and apply two or three times a day.

For Thrush or Canker: Burnt alum, 4 oz.; sulphate of iron, 2 oz.; sulphate of copper, 1 oz.; camphor, 2 drams. Mix.

Blue vitriol, in the proportion of two drams to a pint of water is an excellent application for wounds. If a caustic effect is desired, increase the quantity to an ounce or more, and it will be found a fine preparation to rouse old ulcers to a healthy action.

For a healing ointment the following is unrivalled: 2½ lbs. palm oil, 2 lbs. lard, ½ lb. gum turpentine, ¼ lb. beeswax, 1 lb. calamine. Simmer all together over a slow fire, and it will be fit for use. Put a little in the wound once a day. Wash the wound with warm water and castile soap before applying the ointment.

Wash for Reducing an Inflamed Wound.

One oz. sulphate of zinc, 1 oz. crotus martes, ½ oz. sugar of lead, 1 pint water. A sore will not smell bad when this wash is used.

Wash for Fresh Wounds. A Favorite Remedy of Great Value.

One teaspoonful white vitriol, 1 teaspoonful copperas, 2 teaspoonfuls fine gunpowder; add to 1 quart of boiling water, and let it stand until cool. If the wound is deep, apply with a syringe. One of the best of remedies for the purpose recommended.

Liniment for Open Wounds. A Fine Preparation.

Take sulphate of copper (copperas), 1 oz.; white vitriol, 2 oz.; muriate of soda (salt), 2 oz.; oil linseed, 2 oz.; Orleans molasses, 8 oz. Boil over a slow fire fifteen minutes, in a pint of urine, all of the above ingredients. When nearly cold add 1 oz. of oil of vitriol and 4 oz. spirits of turpentine, and bottle for use. Apply to the wound with a quill, which will soon set the wound to discharging, and perform a cure in a few days. Be careful to keep the wound covered either with a bandage or a plaster. Should be applied once or twice a day until it discharges freely.

Magic Healing Preparation.

Burnt alum, ½ oz.; prepared chalk, 1 oz.; pulverized gum camphor, 1 dram; calamine, pulverized, 2 drams. Mix.

Sprinkle on the sore. Its effect will be apparently wonderful, healing a simple wound in a few hours.

It is well to mention that matter in deep wounds always lodges or runs to the bottom. Hence, in treating such they must be either opened up to the bottom or syringed out carefully. First sponge out with soap and water, then inject the medicine from a syringe. If there is proud flesh, sprinkle on blue vitriol, powdered, or any caustic.

Great latitude is necessary in the treatment of wounds. It is assumed the reader is capable of using some judgment. I give remedies of the greatest value, and if any prudence is shown in their use success must result. I would caution in one respect: do not doctor a wound too much. As a rule, do not dress a wound but once, or at most twice a day.

To Cure an Indolent Ulcer.

Take the green scum that gathers on the water in the frog-ponds in the spring and summer; boil over a slow fire; then add fresh butter to the consistence of an ointment. This is an Indian remedy; cured an ulcer of seventeen years standing that had resisted all other treatment.

Liniment for Foul Ulcers. Good.

Sulphate of copper, 1 oz.; nitric acid, ½ oz.; water, 8 to 12 oz.

Cooling Liniment for External Inflammation. Good.

Goulard extract, 1 oz.; vinegar, 2 oz.; spirits of wine, 3 oz.; water, 1½ pints. Apply with a bandage.

For Inflamed Leg, Galled Shoulders or Back. A Really Good Thing.

Sal ammoniac, 1 oz.; vinegar, 4 oz.; spirits of wine, 2 oz.; tincture arnica, 2 drams; water, ½ pint. Mix, and bathe with it often and thoroughly.

A Very Active Blister.

Two drams corrosive sublimate, 1 oz. lard, ½ oz. tar, 2 drams cantharides. Rub and mix well together. Good for spavins, ringbones, curbs, &c.

Powerful Absorbing Blister.

Equal parts of beniodide of mercury and cantharides, three parts of tar and lard each. Rub in well with the hand for three mornings, and use lard after to soften and take off the scab, when it may be repeated if necessary.

For absorbing enlargements, use beniodide of mercury, one part; from one to three of lard, according to strength desired. One of the finest remedies for the above enlargements.

The following liniment, taken from "Stuart's American Farmer's Horse Book," is highly extolled and used so generally for blistering, counter irritation, spavins, ringbone, splints, curbs, corns, thrush, canker, foot rot or weak heels, bruising of the soles, &c., that I am induced to include it in this part of my work:

Corrosive Liniment.

Take a pint of turpentine, which put in a good strong bottle, adding an ounce of finely pulverized corrosive sublimate and an ounce of gum camphor. Shake well, and let the mixture stand for twenty-four hours, when it will be fit for use.

The value of this liniment depends greatly upon the fineness to which the corrosive sublimate is pulverized. Grind it as fine as possible in a druggist's mortar; pounding with a hammer will not answer. The object of this pulverization is to get the substance in such a form that it will be readily dissolved by the turpentine. There are comparatively few liquids which will dissolve corrosive sublimate, and we claim to have discovered that turpentine is one of these. Corrosive sublimate is well known as one of the most violent poisons. Its combination with turpentine constitutes one of the most powerful of medicines, increasing in its active properties by keeping. We believe it to be the most penetrating liniment in the world. It reaches the seat of disease through any and all obstacles. It destroys all infection, putridity, ulceration, old running sores, proud flesh, and all skin and bone diseases of the horse. It will cure big head and jaw, grease, thrush, scratches, swelled legs, hoof rot, foot evil, corns, ulceration of the foot, (navicular disease,) fistula, poll evil, ringbone and spavin, in their first stages.

In the human subject this liniment has been known to cure repeatedly those troublesome affections known as tetter and scald head; but it is to be used with great caution in these cases, and not at all unless at least ten days old.

Method of using.—Always shake the bottle well before taking out the stopper. Pour the liquid into an earthen vessel, as it corrodes vessels of metal. Apply with a little mop of soft rag. In all bone affections the liniment is to be thoroughly dried in by means of a hot iron held close to the medicated spot, but not close enough to burn the animal. Particular directions are given, in connection with the description of diseases, how to proceed in reference to quantity and manner of using the liniment.

Caution.—Keep the materials for making out of the way of children, as it is a violent poison. Persons unacquainted with it are sometimes alarmed at the severity with which it acts upon the skin of the horse. It inflames, corrodes and puffs out the skin. For cracked heels, spavin, ringbone, curb, windgalls, grease heels and all purposes of counter irritation, Stuart recommends that a little be spread on with a little sponge or mop. For corns, weak heels, tenderness of the feet, a diseased condition of the frog and sole, showing want of healthy secretion, or want of growth, bathe the parts thoroughly with it, and heat in with a shovel, repeating the application once a day. He says it is a specific for big leg if applied once a day.

Note.—This is an active remedy, strongly poisonous.—D. M.

SPRAINS AND BRUISES.

It must be borne in mind, the first object in treating acute inflammation caused by injury of any kind is to lower the inflammation. Cold water, or one ounce of sugar of lead to a pint of water, would be better, and is a remedy of great value, to be used repeatedly until relief is afforded.

The following is excellent: Saltpeter, 4 oz.; sugar of lead, 1 oz.; muriate of ammonia, 1 oz.; common salt, 1 pint; cold water, 2 galls. Mix and bathe the parts affected; or keep constantly wet with the following, which is good: Tincture arnica, 2 oz.; cold water, 1 quart. This will prevent inflammation or swelling following a bruise or sprain.

Anodyne Stimulating Liniment.

Spirits of hartshorn, 1½ oz.; sulphuric ether, 1½ oz.; spirits of turpentine, ½ oz.; sweet oil, ¾ oz.; oil of cloves, ½ oz.; chloroform, 1 oz. Put into a strong 8 ounce bottle and cork tightly; keep in a dark place, or wrap with paper. This liniment relieves pain, and is good for lameness, etc., and for all cases of strains and soreness. To be well rubbed in.

Oil of turpentine, 1 oz.; tinc. opium, 1 oz.; soap liniment, 1 oz.; tinc. capsicum, ½ oz. Stimulating liniment; good for rheumatism, sprains, etc.

Magic Liniment.

Used very generally; good not only for sprains, bruises, etc., after the acute stage, but a fine counter-irritant for pleurisy, inflammation, etc.: Oil of spike, 2 oz.; organum, 2 oz.; hemlock, 2 oz.; wormwood, 2 oz.; sweet oil, 4 oz.; spirits ammonia, 2 oz.; gum camphor, 2 oz.; spirits turpentine, 2 oz.; proof spirits, 1 quart—90 per cent. Mix well together, and bottle tight.

Sweating Liniment for Windgalls, Etc.

Strong mercurial ointment, 2 oz.; camphor, ½ oz.; oil of rosemary, 2 drams; oil of turpentine, 1 oz. Mix.

Very Strong Sweating Blister, for Windgalls, Curbs, Splints, Etc.

Beniodide of mercury, ½ to 1 dram; powdered arnica leaves, 1 dram; soap liniment, 2 oz. Mix.

Very Strong Blister for Spavins, Ringbones, Curbs, Etc.

Finely powdered cantharides, 1 oz.; powdered euphorbium, 2 drams; lard, 1 oz.; tar, 2 oz.

Cough Powder.

Fenugreek, ginger, licorice and bloodroot, equal parts. Half proportion lobelia and camphor may be added. Dose, tablespoonful twice a day. For heaves, add more camphor.

Farcy—Cure of.

One-quarter pound sulphur, ⅛ pound saltpeter, 1 ounce black antimony. If acute, give one tablespoonful twice a day. If sub-acute, once or twice a week.

The sum of $50 was repeatedly paid for this prescription. It is undoubtedly the best preparation ever published for this dangerous disease. Have been informed repeatedly by subscribers of their curing bad cases of farcy by this remedy.

Cracked Heels.

Two ounces resin, 2 ounces copperas, 2 ounces alum, 1 ounce beeswax, 1 pint tar, size hen's egg of tallow; boil over a slow fire, skim off the filth and add the scrapings of sweet elder a handful; when cool, fit for use.

This is a remedy of great value; have used it with the most marked success. This is the best remedy of which the writer has any knowledge for the cure of cracked heels. It is a splendid healing preparation for scratches, saddle or collar galls, or any inflammation of the skin, and is worth many times the price of this book.

Cure of Scratches.

Four ounces tincture arnica, 4 ounces glycerine. If heels are cracked badly, add: 1 ounce iodine, 2 ounces tincture myrrh, ½ ounce gun powder (powdered fine.) Put all into a bottle and shake thoroughly; put on two or three times a day.

In treating scratches, first give a dose of physic, or a few bran mashes.

Cure of Grease Heels.

One-quarter pound bar lead melted, mix in sulphur while hot; let it burn until pulverized. Then add a tablespoonful of hog's lard. Wash the parts and rub on the ointment once or twice a day. A *favorite remedy, and claimed to be very effective.* Given by a physician.

To Reduce Swelling of the Legs and Strengthen the Tendons after Hard Driving.

A favorite remedy on Long Island. One pint alcohol, 1 ordinary sized beef gall, 1 ounce organum, 1 ounce oil of spike, 1 ounce gum myrrh, ½ ounce camphor gum. First wash and rub clean and dry. Then bathe with the liniment and rub dry. Then apply again and bandage the leg, being careful not to bandage too tight.

This is the best liniment for the purpose recommended I have ever used. It should be kept in every stable.

To Recruit a Horse Hide-bound or Otherwise Out of Sorts.

Nitrate potassa (or saltpeter), 4 ounces; crude antimony, 1 ounce; sulphur, 3 ounces. Nitrate of potassa and antimony should be finely pulverized, then add the sulphur and mix the whole well together. Dose: A tablespoonful of the mixture in a bran mash daily, for a week or two. This is my favorite preparation when I wish to get in a condition. Its effect upon a horse out of sorts is sometimes wonderful.

Condition Powders.

Take 1 pound of ginger, 1 ounce of anise seed, pulverized, 1 ounce of fenugreek seed, 2 ounces of ginseng root pulverized, 1 ounce of the seed of sumach berries pulverized, 1 ounce of antimony; mix it with one pound of brown sugar. This is excellent for coughs, colds, or to give a horse an appetite.

To Cure Cough—No. 2. Excellent.

Put all the tar into alcohol it will cut, and add one-third in quantity of tincture belladonna. Dose: From one to two teaspoonfuls once or twice a day. Very good.

To Cure Cough—No. 3.

Take tartar emetic, 1 ounce; resin, 2 ounces; bloodroot, 1 ounce; salts of tartar, 2 ounces; ginger, 2 ounces. Mix, and give a teaspoonful three times a day, in the feed.

For Fresh Strains, Etc.

Carbonate ammonia, 2 ounces; apple vinegar, ½ gill. Rub in well. An excellent remedy.

Preparation to Kill Lice on Horses.

One ounce of arsenic to a pail of soft water. The horse should be washed thoroughly in some warm place. It is not known to many that hen lice and common human body lice grow on horses with great rapidity. This remedy is a sure cure, and is invaluable.

Healing Ointment for Cuts, Galls, Etc. Good.

Oxide of zinc, pulverized fine, 4 drams; carbolic acid, 6 grains; lard, 1 ounce. Melt the lard and stir in the zinc. Add the carbolic acid and mix thoroughly. Apply once or twice a day to the cut or injury. Will cause a healthy discharge from a foul ulcer.

Healing Ointment for Thrush, Saddle Galls, Etc. A Good Thing.

Two ounces blue vitriol, 1 ounce white vitriol, powdered finely as possible and rubbed down with one pound of tar and two pounds of lard.

Opthalmy Simple.

Inflammation of the eyes frequently occurs in young horses soon after stabling.

Symptoms.—A watery discharge from the eye, eyelids partly closed, membrane of lid on under side much reddened.

Treatment.—Give the following ball, and bleed from the angular vein under the eye, allowing it to bleed until it stops from the coagulation of the blood: Barbadoes aloes, 6 drams; nitrate potassa, 2 drams; tartrate of antimony, 1 dram. Mix with molasses or honey in one ball. Bathe the eye with a solution as follows: Laudanum, 1 oz.; rain water, 1 pint; mix. Or: Acetate of lead, 1 dram; sulphate of zinc, ½ dram; rain water, 3 pints. Mix for use. Either of the above may be applied with a soft sponge two or three times a day.

Specific Opthalmy, (Moon Blindness.)

Symptoms.—Membranes of the eye reddened, opacity, or white film over the eyeball, watery discharges from the eyes, which are partially closed. This disease is seldom cured effectually, but the eyes may be cleared up and the attacks warded off for some time by the following treatment: Open the bowels with the following ball: Barbadoes aloes, 1 oz.: gentian, pulverized, 2 drams; niter, pulverized, 2 drams. Mix with molasses for one ball. Give night and morning one-half dram doses of colchicum root in the feed, which should be mashes, and bathe the eye with the following wash: Laudanum, 1 oz.; rain water, 1 pint. Mix, and bathe the eye two or three times a day. Or: Extract belladonna, 1 dram; rain water, 1 pint. Mix and use in like manner.

Eye Wash.

Take three hens' eggs and break them into a quart of clear, cold rain water; stir until a thorough mixture is effected; boil over a slow fire, stirring every few minutes; add half an ounce of sulphate of zinc, (white vitriol;) continue the boiling a short time, and the compound is ready for use. In this preparation a solid substance, or curd, is precipitated or thrown down, and a liquid solution rests upon the top. This is the best wash for the sore eyes of either man or beast that was ever made. The curd applied to the inflamed eye at night will draw the fever and soreness nearly all out by morning. After two or three days the water should be strained from the curd and put into a bottle for future use. This eye wash is invaluable. No physician or druggist has ever discovered a medicine of the kind equal to it. When applied to the human eye it should be diluted.

Hoof Liniment for Contracted or Sore Feet. One of the Very Best Remedies.

Venice turpentine, ½ pint; aqua ammonia, 2 oz; salts of niter, 1 oz.; benzine, 1 oz.; alcohol, 3 oz. Apply to the edge of the hair and all over the hoof once a day for a week; after that, for a week or two, three or four times a week, as may be necessary.

Grease Heels.

This is a white, offensive, greasy discharge from the heels of the horse. The skin becomes hot, tender and swollen. The acrid character of the discharge often causes large portions of the skin to slough away, leaving an ugly sore behind.

Treatment.—Open the bowels with the following ball: Barbadoes aloes, 1 oz.; pulverized gentian root, 2 drams; pulverized ginger, 1 dram; water sufficient to make the ball. Wash the parts well, and poultice for two or three days with the following: Flax seed meal mixed with a solution of 2 drams sulphate of zinc to a pint of water, which keep clean, and bathe frequently with glycerine, or the solution of zinc; or a solution of the chloride of lime may be used; or the bichloride of mercury may be used in inveterate cases with good results, provided it is not repeated oftener than once a week.

Thrush.

This is a rotting of the frog, with a discharge of matter from the cleft or division of the frog, occasionally producing lameness. The treatment is simple and effectual. Wash the parts well with soap and water, then apply powdered sulphate of copper to the parts, and fill up all the cavities with cotton, packed in so as to keep out all dirt. This process should be repeated in a few days if necessary.

Canker.

This is a more aggravated form of thrush, often proving very troublesome to manage. It is a continuation of the thrush between the horny frog and the internal structures of the foot, causing separation between them.

Treatment.—Cut away all the horn which has been separated from the soft structures of the foot, and apply the following ointment: Take equal parts of pine tar and lard, melt over a slow fire, and add sulphuric acid very slowly until ebullition (boiling) ceases. Or use: Collodion, ½ oz.; castor oil, 1 oz. Mix and apply to the parts. The foot must be protected from dirt by a bandage or a leathern boot.

Warts.

These fungous growths appear in the horse most frequently about the mouth, nose and lips, but they are occasionally found upon other parts of the body. They are sometimes found in large numbers about the lips of colts, and are generally rubbed off or drop off. If, however, they grow large and become deeply rooted, they may be cut off by passing a needle through the center, armed with a double thread, and tied tightly around the neck on each side. This prevents the possibility of the ligatures being rubbed off. Or they may be painted over with the per-manganate of potash, a few applications of which will entirely destroy warts of a large size; or they may be removed with a knife.

Profuse Staling.

The causes of this disease are, the improper use of diuretic medicines, as saltpeter, resin, &c. Unwholesome food will sometimes produce it.

Treatment.—Give one of the following balls every night: Powdered opium, ½ oz.; powdered kino, 1 oz.; prepared chalk, 1 oz. Mix with molasses, and make six balls.

Bloody Urine

Is generally the result of injuries of the loins, unwholesome food, violent exercise, &c.

Treatment.—Give plenty linseed tea to drink; if the animal refuses it, drench him. Give internally, once a day, one of the following pills: Sugar of lead, 1 oz.; linseed meal, 2 oz. Mix with molasses, and divide into eight parts.

Quitter.

This is a formation of pus between the hoof and the soft structure within; a sore at the coronet or upper part of the foot, which at first is a hard, smooth tumor, soon becoming soft, and breaks, discharging quantities of pus.

Treatment.—Poultice the foot for several days with flax seed meal. As soon as the hoof becomes soft, cut away all loose portions, but no more, and inject with a syringe either of the following once a day: Chloride of zinc, 2 drams, dissolved in a pint of water; or, sulphate of zinc, 1½ drams, in a pint of water; or, nitrate of silver, 2 drams, in a pint of water; or glycerine may be used with advantage. Before using the wash have the foot well cleaned with castile soap and water.

Mange.

Take the horse in the sun and scrub him thoroughly all over with castile soap and water, then wash him well from head to tail with gas water, in which put 2 drams white hellebore to the gallon. He must now be put in another stall, distant from the one in which he has been standing. Thus treated, it rarely requires more than one washing to effect a permanent cure. The harness should be thoroughly scrubbed and put away for six or eight weeks. These precautions are necessary to success in this otherwise troublesome disease.

No. 2.—Oil turpentine, 4 oz.; oil tar, 4 oz.; linseed oil, 6 oz. Mix.

A Shoulder Strain.

This is caused by severe blows, strains or falls, &c.

Symptoms.—The animal drags the leg, with the toe on the ground, and cannot raise the foot.

Treatment.—Local bleeding is very effectual, with a purging ball. Fomenting the shoulder with hot water will be found useful in two or three days. The following liniment should be applied two or three times a day: Laudanum, 1 oz.; spirits camphor, 1 oz.; tincture myrrh, 1 oz.; castile soap, 1 oz.; alcohol, 1 pint. Mix for use. Or: Linseed oil, 1 pint; oil turpentine, 2 oz.; spirits hartshorn, 3 oz. Mix, shake well, and use once a day for three or four days.

Nasal Gleet.

This is a chronic discharge from one or both nostrils, of a whitish, muco-purulent matter, the result usually of neglected catarrh. The general health of the animal does not seem to suffer; he looks well, feeds well and works well, yet we have this discharge, which is caused by weakness in the secretory vessels of the lining membrane of the nose.

The successful treatment in all cases where this disorder has existed has been on the tonic principle. Bleeding and purging are positively injurious. Give one of the following powders night and morning: Seaquin-chloride of iron, 2 oz.; powdered cinnamon, 1 oz. Mix and divide into four powders. Or: Carbonate of iron, pulverized gentian and pulverized quassia, of each 1 oz. Divide into four powders. Or: Nux vomica, pulverized, ½ oz.; linseed meal, 2 oz. Divide into eight powders. Another good preparation is: Muriate of Barytes, ½ oz.; linseed meal, 1 oz. Divide into eight powders.

Caustics

Are substances which burn away the tissues of the body by decomposition of their elements, and are valuable to destroy fungus growth and set up healthy action.

Corrosive sublimate, in powder, acts energetically.

Nitrate of silver is excellent to lower granulation.

Sulphate of copper, not so strong as the above, but good.

Chloride of zinc is a powerful caustic. It may be used in sinuses, in solution, 7 drams in a pint of water.

Milder Caustics.

Verdigris, either in powder or mixed with lard, as an ointment, in proportion of one to three.

Butter of Antimony.—For corns, canker, indisposition of the sole to secrete healthy horn, wounds in the foot not attended by healthy action, and for every case where the superficial application of a caustic is needed, the chloride of antimony (butter of antimony) is one of the very best.

Sticking-Plaster, for Cuts or Wounds.

Burgundy pitch, 4 oz.; tallow, 2 oz. Melt the articles together, and spread on linen or cloth while hot. Cut in strips of proper length and width, and draw the wound together; warm the strips and apply them. Clip the hair short where the plaster is to be applied.

To Abate Swelling Caused by an Injury.

Take common wormwood, 2 oz.; New England Rum, 1 quart. Steep the wormwood in the liquor and apply thoroughly.

I enclose the following receipt as one of reputed great value for the cure of RINGBONES and SPAVINS. Will take off the enlargement. One hundred dollars could not buy this recipe, and the owner deemed himself in possession of the best remedy in the world. It is one of the best of this class of remedies.

Ringbone Liniment.

First.—Alcohol, 14 oz.; iodine, 304 grains; bichloride of mercury, 150 grains. Let stand in a sand bath twenty-two hours, then add 230 drops croton oil; let stand in sand bath twenty-two hours longer, then bottle for use.

Powder for Spavins and Ringbones.

Quicksilver, 14 oz.; nitric acid, 7 oz.; stir one minute; cantharides, 7 drams; stir five minutes; sulphuric acid, 7 oz.; stir three minutes; 50 drops of the above liniment. Let stand five hours, stir every half hour, then add 7 oz. prepared chalk.

First shave the hair off the "bunch," then apply the liniment with a lather brush. Sprinkle a little of the powder on paper, and rub on, after washing with the liniment. When the bunch is reduced two-thirds, wash with warm water and castile soap. In twenty-four hours grease.

This will cure, but it is sure to blemish.

CONTENTS.

www.ingramcontent.com/pod-product-compliance
Lightning Source LLC
LaVergne TN
LVHW021407110826
845150LV00007B/1815

* 9 7 8 1 4 2 5 5 1 2 1 5 6 *